Clinical Suc[illegible]

in

Management of Advanced Periodontitis

Roger Detienville, DDS
Assistant Professor
Department of Periodontics
School of Dental Surgery
René Descartes University-Paris 5
Paris, France

English Translation by
Nicolai Johnson, DDS
Private Practice
Paris, France

Quintessence International

quintessence books

Paris, Chicago, Berlin, Tokyo, London, Milan, Barcelona,
Istanbul, São Paulo, New Delhi, Moscow, Prague, and Warsaw

First published in French in 2002 by Quintessence International, Paris
Le Traitement des Parodontites Sévères

To Monique

Quintessence International
11 bis, Rue d'Aguesseau
75008 Paris
France

Design: STDI, Lassay-les-Châteaux, France
Printing and Binding: EMD, Lassay-les-Châteaux, France

Printed in France

Acknowledgments

I would like to acknowledge the colleagues listed below:

Salima Benmehdi
Claire Boski
Alain Canac
Fabrice Chérel
Michel Degrange
Cédric Fiévet
Bernard Fleiter
Dominique Guez
Alain Lautrou
Thierry Perronnet
Philippe Rajzbaum
Franck Renouard
Thierry Taïeb
Jean-François Tulasne

For their valuable help and dedication, I would also like to thank Jean-Louis Giovannoli and Jean-Marie Korbendau

Table of Contents

Severity of Periodontal Disease

1

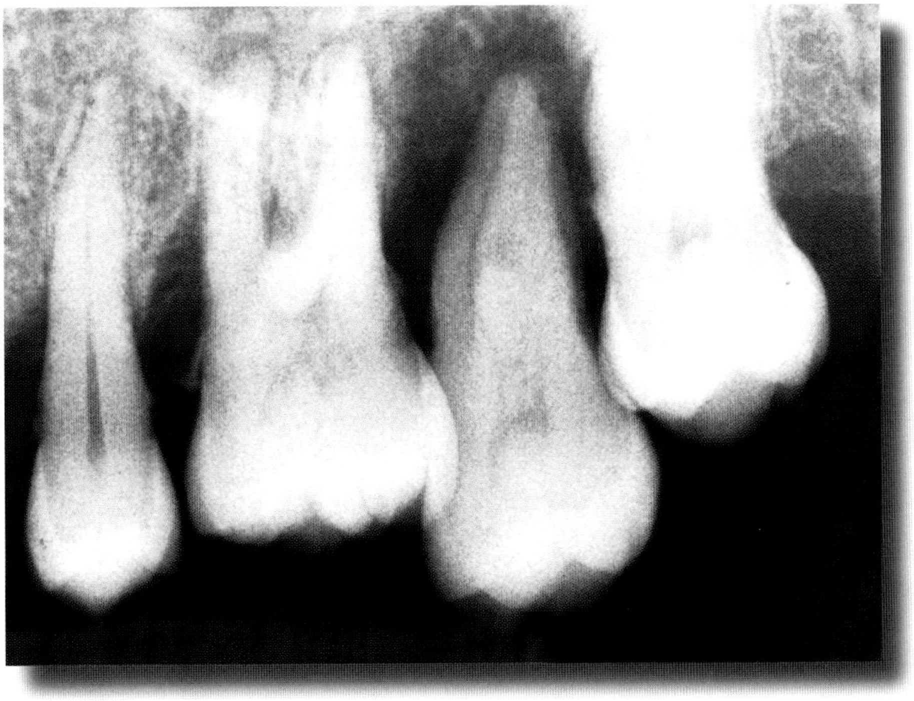

Severity Criteria

Periodontal disease is an inflammatory disease caused by a bacterial infection. It is characterized by a progressive destruction of the dental attachment tissues. Left untreated, it may lead to complete loss of dental attachment structures and subsequently loss of teeth.

The primary objective of treatment is to arrest the progressive destruction of periodontal tissue and thus to arrest loss of attachment structures. However, the infectious process involved in periodontal disease is complex. Host susceptibility and the presence of pathogenic bacterial species, whether exogenous or commensal, interact and either promote or hinder the progression of the disease. Simultaneously, numerous local or environmental factors exert an influence on the etiologic agents and the course of disease. Because of its multifactorial nature, periodontal disease is difficult to manage. In formulating treatment strategies, both the patient's periodontal susceptibility and the amount of periodontal destruction need to be taken into account. Repair and regeneration have become realistic objectives in the current context of periodontal therapeutics. For this reason, a methodic assessment of severity factors is a crucial step in treatment planning.

Severe periodontal disease is characterized by:

- Destruction of periodontal attachment tissue exceeding one third of the root's length
- Class II or III furcation invasion
- Probing depths exceeding 6 mm
- Attachment loss exceeding 4 mm

Some teeth have already been lost or are unlikely to be maintained. The indication of prosthetic restorations for the replacement of missing teeth denotes the irreversible aspect of treatment in the periodontal patient. However, prosthetic rehabilitation may seem a risky endeavor in the context of uncontrolled periodontal disease. This raises several questions concerning both the disease itself and the global treatment strategy:

- Is infection control possible in all forms of periodontitis?
- Are there severity factors? How can they be detected? Can they be eliminated?
- What are the risk factors?
- What would be the best treatment strategy?
- To what extent can a conservative approach be applied?
- What are the different criteria that indicate the decision to extract?
- When should the decision to extract be made?
- What is the prognosis for the remaining teeth?
- Is it possible to place implants in the context of advanced periodontal disease?
- Should we carry out periodontal treatments less often and place implants more often?
- What are the optimal conditions for successful therapy?

In the 1990s, the strategy consisting of root debridement with scaling and planing with or without surgical techniques and followed by periodontal maintenance every 3 to 6 months was considered the best treatment for the majority of periodontal diseases (Goodson 1994). However, the so-called refractory forms emerged; these were characterized by poor response to treatment (Figs 1-1a and 1-1b). In these specific cases, antibiotic therapy was recommended. Since then, however, progress in microbiologic knowledge no longer limits the use of antibiotic therapy to the refractory forms of periodontal disease. Taken together, these elements demonstrate the need for a sound understanding of the complex microbiology of periodontal disease in clinical practice.

A better understanding of the etiology and pathogenesis of periodontal diseases has allowed for the development of new guidelines for management and treatment; this represents a major step toward carrying out treatment strategies better suited to individual patients. An increasingly specific approach, taking into account factors such as patient susceptibility, features of periodontal infection, and individual severity factors, will no doubt lead to a reduction of the number of refractory forms and lay out a clinical context favorable to tissue response.

The American Academy of Periodontology's 2000 classification now serves as a reference. Periodontal disease treatments should be carried out in accordance with the diagnostic criteria specified in this classification. Advanced periodontitis is most often observed in younger patients, though it does not represent a distinct clinical subset; it is observed in chronic and aggressive forms of periodontal disease, both of which represent the principal subunits of the new classification. In the case of chronic periodontitis, treatment is relatively straightforward: the infection is characterized by a significant amount of plaque buildup and features a predominant commensal bacterial population with local aggravating factors. In the case of aggressive periodontitis, a more specific protocol must take into account the involvement of a more complex bacterial flora, specific patient susceptibility factors, and additional risk factors. Here again, formulating a precise diagnosis is a crucial step in patient management.

Defining treatment success in periodontal practice represents a difficult task. It implies both complete elimination of infectious processes and associated inflammation as well as durable prevention of recurrence in all previously pathologic periodontal sites. Infection control is the key to success, though it is the aspect of treatment that is most difficult to accomplish. The ultimate goal is durable restoration, both esthetic and functional, while attempting to avoid the use of partial dentures.

Currently, there is a strong incentive toward the application of evidence-based solutions and techniques. However, statistical analysis is more difficult to carry out in the clinical setting than in the context of pure research. Clinical practice can therefore demonstrate its efficacy and ultimately point out elements of scientific truth through interpretation of scientific information.

Among these indicators of clinical proof are the following:

- Continuous, progressive loss of periodontal support is a significant and undesirable clinical proof.
- Durable elimination of clinical signs of inflammation and long-term maintenance of periodontal support structures are significant positive clinical proofs.
- Attachment gain and reduced probing depths are significant, ideal clinical parameters that indicate long-term clinical success.

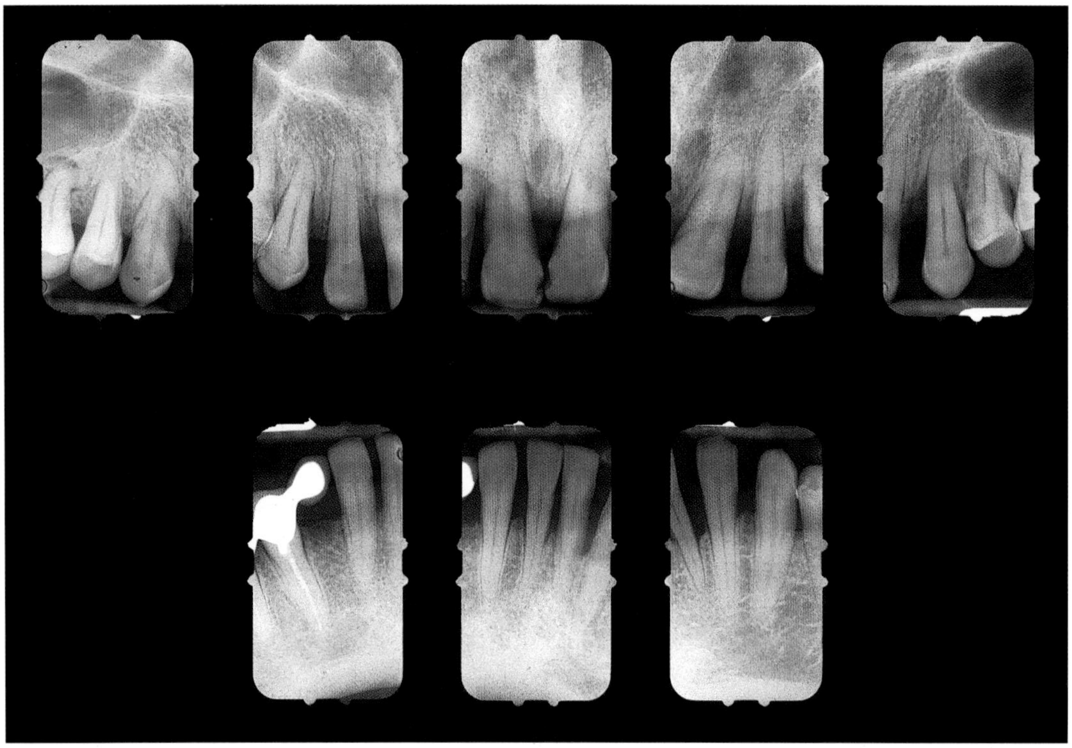

Fig 1-1a Aggressive periodontitis in a 40-year-old woman who is subject to stress and smokes one pack of cigarettes a day. The patient experienced an emotional shock 5 years earlier. A conventional treatment plan was initiated and included periodontal surgery throughout all quadrants. Professional maintenance (scaling and root planing) was carried out every 3 months, and the patient responded well.

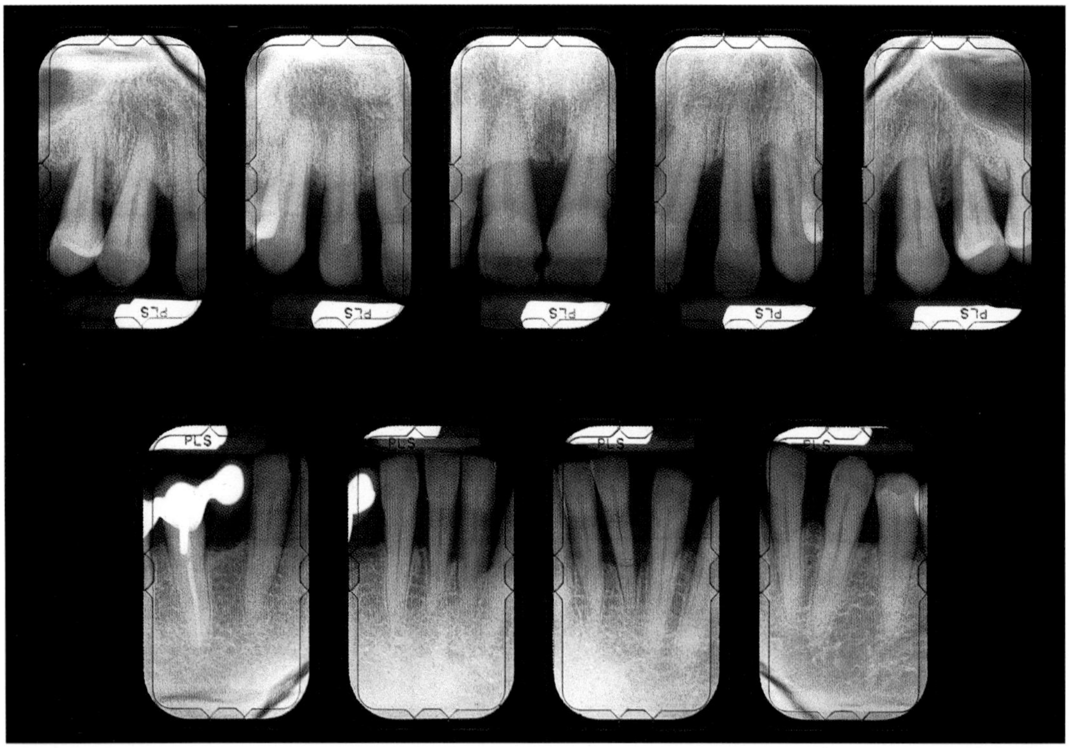

Fig 1-1b Four years after treatment and maintenance therapy. Periodontal status has deteriorated in all areas. Observe the new attachment losses, dental migrations, and larger diastemata. It is clear that periodontal disease is not controlled. This patient's disease was refractory to conventional treatment. Specific risk factors in this patient were underestimated.

Prevalence of Periodontal Disease

Periodontal disease predominantly affects the adult population. The overall prevalence of periodontitis is high. According to some authors, 90% of the general population have signs of periodontitis and 50% of individuals aged 15 to 19 years have at least one periodontal pocket (Waerhaug 1975; Sheiham 1978). An analysis of the natural history of the disease is informative and shows that there are several periodontal disease subtypes.

A first longitudinal study, carried out in a tea-picking community of Sri Lanka (Loë et al 1986), studied a group of individuals who were relatively well isolated from dental care over a period of 15 years. At the end of the study, the authors defined three groups:

- The first group represented 8% of all studied individuals and was characterized by the presence of a rapidly progressing form of periodontal disease. Approximately 20 teeth had been lost for periodontal reasons before the age of 40 years, and all teeth were generally lost at the age of 45 years (Figs 1-2a and 1-2b).
- The second group represented 81% of all studied individuals; this group featured a moderate form of periodontitis and an average of 7 teeth lost for periodontal reasons at age 45 years (Figs 1-3a and 1-3b).
- The third group represented 11% of the study group and was characterized by the absence of periodontitis; no teeth were lost to periodontal disease, and despite the presence of gingivitis, no evidence of periodontal destruction was observed (Figs 1-4a and 1-4b).

The results of this study were confirmed in other population groups. This distribution is considered valid in various populations, regardless of geographic localization.

In Western Europe, a study of nonedentulous individuals aged 45 to 54 years showed that 36% presented with a severe form of periodontitis, 31.9% had a moderate form of periodontal disease, and 32% presented no signs or symptoms of periodontal destruction (Ainamo et al 1982). It is noteworthy that edentulous cases were not taken into account. In France, according to a study by the Institut National de la Santé et de la Recherche Médicale (INSERM), 90% of the general population presents with various degrees of periodontal pathology (INSERM 1999).

In Sweden, 13% of individuals examined in 1973 and reexamined between 1988 and 1991 displayed signs of advanced periodontal disease with bone loss of more than 20% in more than six anatomic sites. Most frequently involved were maxillary (18%) and mandibular (12.8%) premolars followed by maxillary first molars (13.5%). Risk factors associated with disease progression were also stated: presence of supragingival plaque, number of probing depths exceeding 4 mm at baseline, smoking, age, heredity, stress, sociologic factors, and presence of systemic disease (Norderyd et al 1999).

In a study carried out in the United States (Brown et al 1989). The authors reported that 15% of the investigated population presented no sign of periodontal disease and that 50% had gingivitis with no evidence of periodontitis. Moderate periodontitis, with probing depths between 4 and 6 mm, was found in 33% of the group. Advanced periodontitis, featuring probing depths exceeding 6 mm, was observed in 8% of patients and involved one to two teeth. Terminal periodontal destruction leading to tooth extraction was observed in only 4% of studied cases. Easy access to dental care and hygiene practices, and living in an economically advanced country, all reduce the prevalence of periodontitis.

A more recent study performed in the United States showed that approximately 35% of adults present signs of periodontal disease. They represent more than 60 million individuals, among which 12.6% have an aggressive form of periodontitis. Prevalence increases in males and in African American and Mexican communities (Albandar et al 1999).

In a study carried out in urban communities in the United States, Craig et al (2001) compared the prevalence of periodontitis in three distinct ethnic groups—Asian American, African American, and Hispanic American. The authors reported higher prevalence and severity of periodontitis in the African American community. This is correlated to limited access to private dental care and a higher smoking rate. Overall, clinical signs of periodontal disease are found to be more advanced in low-income households.

In conclusion, among individuals presenting with bacterial plaque and calculus due to poor plaque control:

- 8% to 15% are likely to develop an aggressive form of periodontal disease that will probably compromise their dentition in the absence of periodontal management.
- 60% of these individuals are likely to develop a moderate level of periodontal damage.
- 15% to 30% present no periodontal destruction despite the presence of gingivitis.
- Gingivitis does not always evolve toward periodontitis.
- Low socioeconomic indices, as well as certain biologic risk factors, seem to increase the risk for developing an aggressive form of periodontitis.

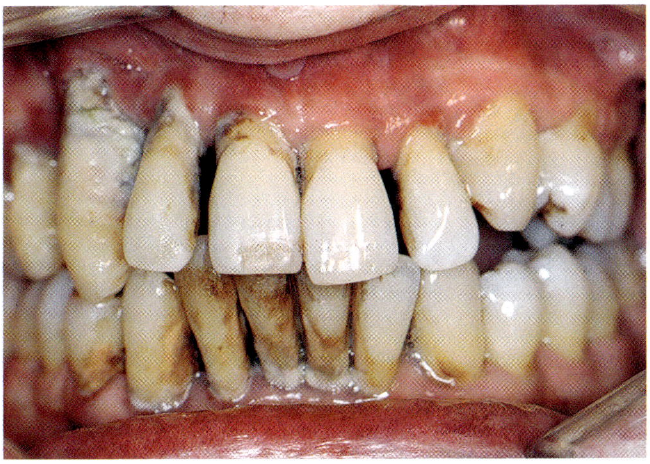

Fig 1-2a Aggressive periodontitis in a 50-year-old man. There is significant functional impairment; all teeth are mobile.

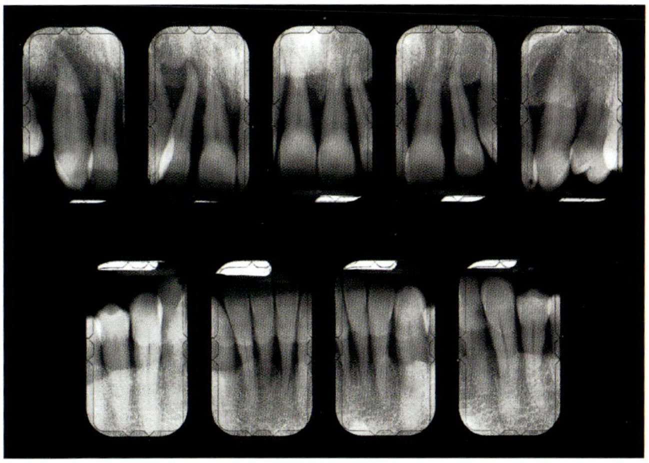

Fig 1-2b Destruction and attachment losses exceed 9 mm.

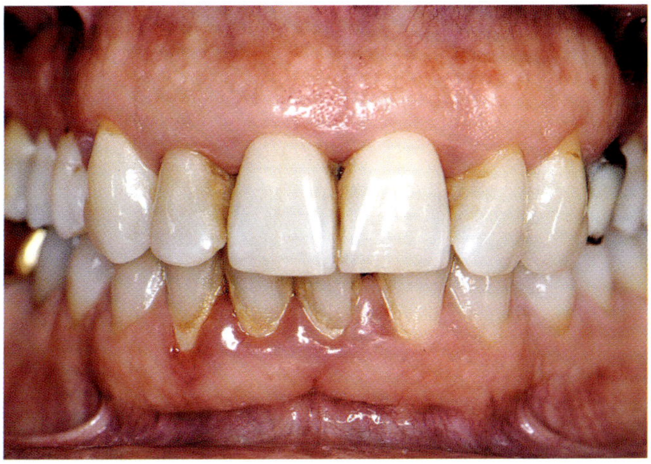

Fig 1-3a In this 40-year-old patient, periodontitis is moderate.

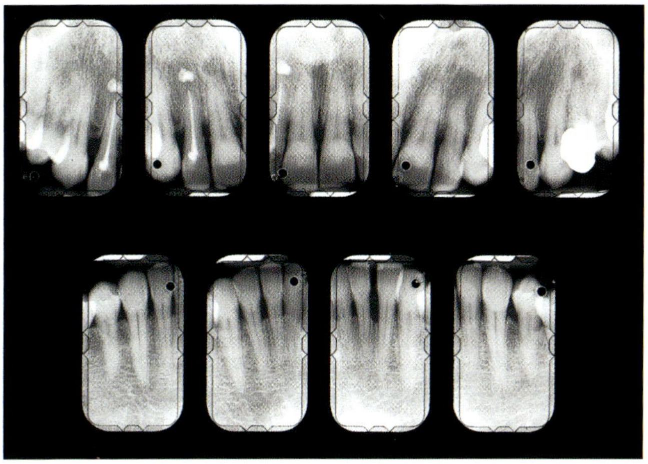

Fig 1-3b Destruction and attachment losses are evenly distributed throughout the dentition and are less than 30%.

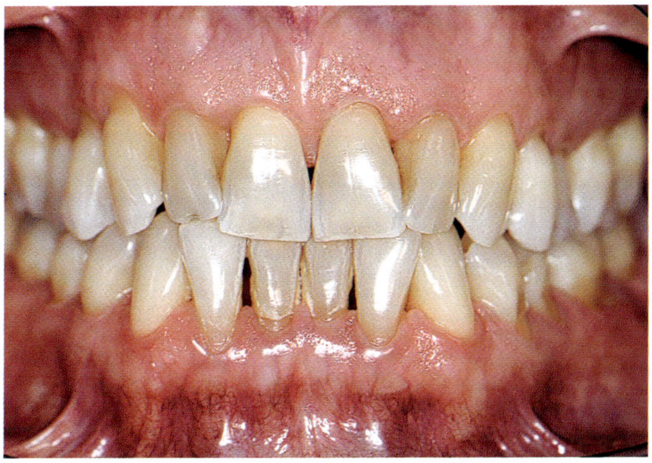

Fig 1-4a This 77-year-old patient presents no sign of periodontitis, despite the absence of preventive care.

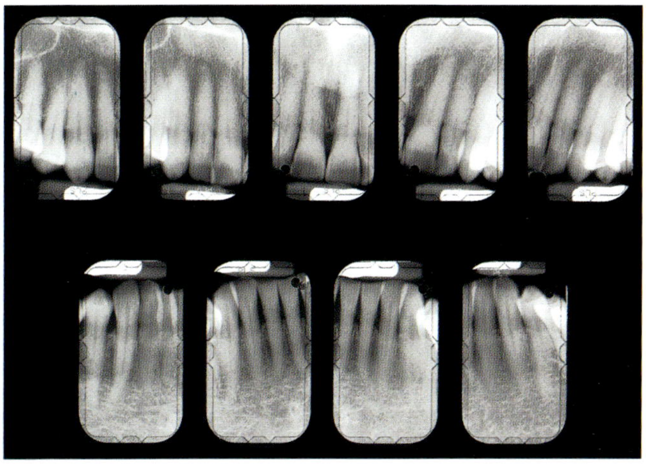

Fig 1-4b There is no evidence of periodontal destruction.

Pathogenesis of Periodontal Disease

2

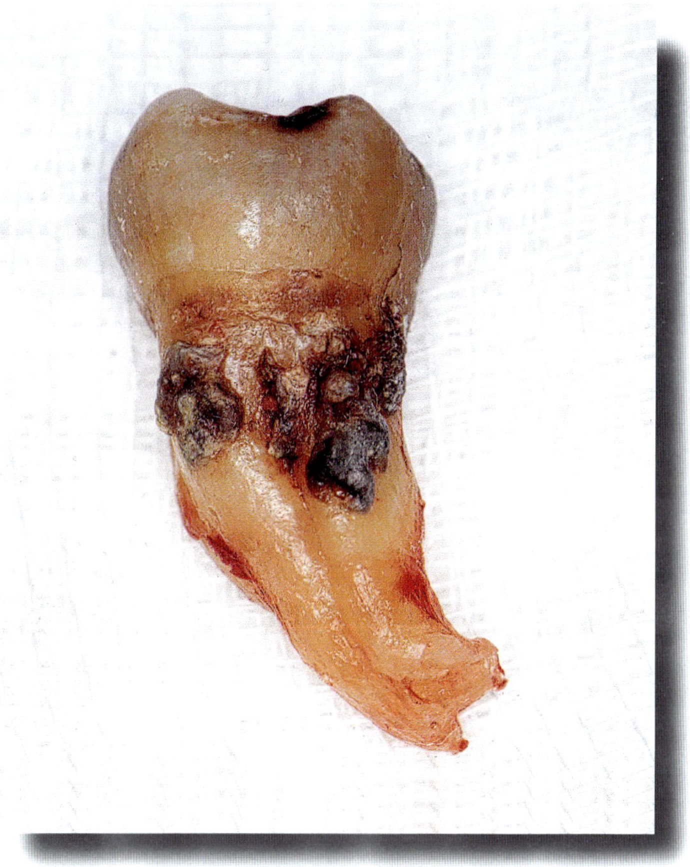

Periodontal disease is an infectious disease caused by the presence of bacterial plaque (Timmerman et al 2001). Bacterial plaque is a nonmineralized accumulation of microbes that is able to adhere firmly to dental, restorative, and prosthetic surfaces. Bacterial plaque has been found to have structural organization. It cannot be displaced by mouth rinsing or by a high-pressure water spray (Listgarten 1994). Its growth is regulated by a dynamic balance between the oral microbiota and a number of factors that may either promote or inhibit the development of specific bacterial populations. Supragingival plaque essentially contains aerobic bacteria. In subgingival plaque, the proportion of gram-negative anaerobes increases.

Different forms of periodontitis have different bacteriologic etiologies. Features of periodontal disease are also determined by factors that modify host response or those that modulate individual host susceptibility, whether systemic, genetic, environmental, or acquired. These modifiers can activate or inhibit mechanisms involved in host response.

The protagonists of the response to bacterial insult are normally involved in tissue protection, but they also may be involved in the processes resulting in tissue destruction. This means that an episode of tissue regeneration may follow an episode of tissue destruction. From a treatment standpoint, this justifies the use of conservative techniques that utilize the potential for repair and regeneration, rather than using more aggressive, irreversible approaches in treating periodontal disease.

Biofilms and Bacterial Complexes

Three bacterial species seem to be involved in most forms of periodontal disease (except in necrotizing ulcerative periodontitis): *Porphyromonas gingivalis*, *Actinobacillus actinomycetemcomitans*, and *Tannerella forsythensis* (formerly *Bacteroides forsythus*). Intrafamilial transmission is possible and seems to be associated with individual susceptibility factors. When these bacterial forms are present, all the infected members of a given family carry the same clonal type. Usually, this same clonal type occurs in a given pocket, family member, and family (Socransky and Haffajee 1994). This has multiple consequences in formulating strategies for prevention and treatment.

Two fundamental features of bacterial plaque explain the difficulty in controlling its growth and eliminating it. First, subgingival plaque is organized as a *biofilm* and, second, the bacterial species it harbors interact specifically to form *bacterial complexes*.

The biofilm is formed by the association of bacterial populations adhering to one another or to the surfaces found in their vicinity (Costerton et al 1994). Its specific features account for the resistance of bacterial plaque to the host's usual defense mechanisms (Page et al 1997). Ecologic communities develop and contribute to the survival of the entire host of bacterial populations. Several types of cooperation take place inside these bacterial populations.

Biofilms are resistant to the host's defense mechanisms and to the action of antimicrobial agents.

The gingival crevicular fluid has been shown to contain consistent levels of the molecular components of the complement, high levels of immunoglobulins and of the cellular blood constituents, including leukocytes and polymorphonuclear neutrophils; these systems are all involved in the control and prevention of infectious processes. The gingival crevicular fluid is found in periodontal pockets and therefore lies in close contact with the biofilm. However, bacterial populations resist and thrive; they are able to spread laterally and apically along the root surfaces, causing tissue destruction and an increase in pocket depth.

Like all other biofilms, subgingival microbial plaque is surprisingly resistant and difficult to eradicate. Through the mutual protection they provide to one another, bacterial populations achieve abnormal resistance to the effects of antibiotics and other antimicrobial agents, whether applied locally or administered systemically.

Mechanical debridement is the only efficacious means for disorganizing the biofilm. This is why the combination of scaling and root planing represents a remarkably efficient technique in the treatment of periodontal disease, prior even to any pharmacologic attempt at controlling infection.

The different bacterial species interact by facilitating or inhibiting the progression of periodontal disease. They form bacterial complexes. An understanding of the relations between these bacteria is necessary to further comprehend the biologic features of subgingival plaque and to formulate coherent strategies for plaque control. Among these species, there is a limited number of pathogenic types and a significant number of saprophytic bacteria. Some are exogenous, while others are normally present in dental plaque (Socransky et al 1998). Socransky et al proposed a classification system that attributes four bacterial complexes to distinct color categories, and it has since become a reference.

A actinomycetemcomitans is an exogenous pathogenic microorganism, which means that it is not considered part of the commensal flora. It is a gram-negative facultative anaerobic rod. This microbe is associated with aggressive, localized forms of periodontitis—previously called localized juvenile periodontitis—as well as with generalized periodontitis.

Red complex: *Porphyromonas gingivalis, Treponema denticola, Tannerella forsythensis*

These exogenous species are found in great numbers in subgingival plaque, deep pockets, and advanced lesions. They invade periodontal tissues and the cementum and produce proteolytic enzymes. The different species belonging to this complex, including *A actinomycetemcomitans*, which has not been classified within any complex, are all found within active periodontopathic lesions.

P gingivalis is an exogenous, strictly anaerobic gram-negative rod. It is predominantly found in the gingival sulcus. It is known to alter the local response of neutrophils recruited through inflammatory processes. Many virulence factors are produced by bacterial pathogens and have been studied extensively (Ishikawa et al 1997).

These toxins are harmful to leukocytes. Bacteria-derived lipopolysaccharides promote and maintain tissue destruction. Other bacterial by-products modify both immune response and cell growth–regulating mechanisms. Finally, bacterial proteases induce tissue destruction and cause damage to the components of host immune response—specific antibodies and complement-activating compounds. However, none of these factors considered alone seems to play a decisive role in the pathogenesis of periodontal disease.

On the other hand, rapid development of pathogenic microorganisms such as *P gingivalis* in the subgingival flora seems to have many consequences: this microorganism plays an important role in the organization of the biofilm and in colonization of host tissues; it also promotes growth of other bacterial populations. By neutralizing the initial phase of the acute inflammatory response, *P gingivalis* alters the host's response potential to infection. It therefore promotes not only its own growth but also that of other bacterial species found in the biofilm. For these reasons, *P gingivalis* is commonly found in sites displaying active periodontal tissue destruction (Darveau et al 1997).

The host develops a humoral response to these periodontopathic microorganisms. Screening for specific antibodies produced in response to bacterial infection is now possible and has proved a powerful tool for clinical evaluation and diagnosis.

Several working hypotheses, proposed by Ebersole and Taubman in 1994, have been confirmed:

- Elevated antibody titers produced in response to specific subgingival pathogens reflect the composition of local gingival microbiota.
- Microorganisms identified through high antibody titers are found in the flora of active destruction sites.
- The relation between colonization and specific response is comparable to the processes involved in specific infectious disease.
- The host's systemic response may help to understand etiologic agents as well as risk factors contributing to the initiation and progression of periodontal disease.

Recent studies have shown that periodontal pathogens can be found in individuals whose periodontium is healthy, in other oral areas such as supragingivally and on oral mucosa (Haffajee and Socransky 1994).

However, prolonged presence of pathogenic species in periodontal pockets carries a high likelihood of developing an active phase of periodontal disease. Screening for these bacteria allows for more efficient treatment and better prevention of recurrence. This justifies using culture methods and sensitivity testing in numerous clinical situations, even if the total bacterial load is significantly reduced after root scaling and planing.

Orange complex: *Fusobacterium nucleatum, Prevotella intermedia, Prevotella nigriscens, Peptostreptococcus micros, Campylobacter rectus*

This complex is frequently associated with the red complex mentioned earlier. *Prev intermedia* is systematically associated with *F nucleatum* in deep pockets. Both of these endogenous pathogenic, anaerobic gram-negative microorganisms are responsible for opportunistic commensal infections. *P micros* and *C rectus* are frequently found in sites related to mobile teeth. *P intermedia*, *C rectus*, and *P micros* are frequently observed in the saliva of patients with advanced periodontitis. These bacterial species also have been found to be involved in nonperiodontal infections, including radicular or cutaneous infections. Metronidazole effectively suppresses these bacterial species.

Yellow complex and green complex: *Eikenella corrodens, Actinobacillus actinomycetemcomitans phenotype a, Streptococcus sanguis*

These pathogens are seldom found associated with those belonging to the orange and red complexes. There is probably an antagonistic relation between these subgroups: coexistence of species from the red or orange groups with species from this group is difficult or impossible. This implies that an environment selective for one group is less selective for the other. The so-called beneficial species are found in this group.

Conditions for the Development of Periodontal Disease

The presence of pathogenic bacteria is a necessary though not sufficient condition for the initiation of periodontal disease (Socransky and Haffajee 1992). Several factors have been shown to be required for periodontal disease activation:

- Host susceptibility factors
- Presence of pathogenic agents
- Presence of pathogens that produce virulence factors in amounts exceeding a threshold tolerable to the host
- Absence of beneficial bacterial species
- A favorable environment

From a microbiologic point of view, healthy periodontal tissue can be differentiated from pathologic periodontal tissue by the balance existing between beneficial and pathogenic bacterial species. Healthy periodontium features high rates of beneficial bacteria and low-to-nonexistent pathogenic bacteria counts. On the other hand, pathologic periodontal tissue is characterized by high pathogenic microbe counts that exceed the host's threshold for infection control. Though pathogenic bacterial populations do exist in healthy periodontal tissue, elevated pathogen loads are usually associated with the presence of an active periodontal disease process.

Beneficial + *Pathogenic*	*Beneficial* + ***Pathogenic***
Health	***Disease***

First, total bacterial load should be taken into account.

From a clinical standpoint, the manifestations and the severity level of periodontal disease are determined by complex interactions between microbial infection and host response. Genetic, environmental, and "acquired" factors, such as smoking, stress, and systemic disease, all influence host response (Page et al 1997). These factors are collectively called *risk factors*.

Taken together, these considerations emphasize the importance, when formulating a treatment strategy, of a sound understanding of subgingival microbiology and the ecologic relations existing therein. Aggressive antimicrobial therapy does not respect these therapeutic principles. Microbiologic analyses are very useful, but they can by no means replace a sound appreciation of clinical signs—inflammation and periodontal destruction.

Periodontal Infection

When the delicate balance between the host and the parasitic populations it harbors is broken, microbial invasion surpasses the host's ability to defend itself, and a bacterial infection starts.

During an opportunistic infection, endogenous bacteria induce an infection in an individual whose local or systemic immune status is altered. Most potentially pathogenic bacterial populations are endogenous; therefore, treatment goals are to reduce total bacterial load while facilitating host response. This pathophysiologic model generally applies to chronic periodontitis.

On the other hand, exogenous bacteria, such as *A actinomycetemcomitans* or *P gingivalis*, can induce true infection. The first treatment objective is to eradicate these bacterial populations. This infection type is frequent in aggressive forms of periodontitis.

In advanced forms of periodontitis, both types of infection usually coexist.

In situations where bacteria invade periodontal tissues (*P gingivalis* or *A Actinomycetemcomitans*, for example) antibiotic therapy should be administered, but usually this is done only after initial mechanical treatment has been performed. Otherwise, there is a strong chance for bacterial recolonization of the periodontal pocket.

Host-Bacteria Interactions and Pathogenesis of Periodontal Disease

At the onset of gingival inflammation, all the protagonists of the pathogenesis of periodontitis come into play. These include junctional epithelial cells, numerous leukocytes and their by-products, a great variety of messengers that act as mediators between cellular protagonists, and molecules responsible for tissue destruction (Kornman et al 1997). This cascade of cellular, vascular, and tissue events settles in progressively while bacterial invasion develops. Here again, there seems to be a balance between the actions of proinflammatory substances leading to tissue destruction and the action of compounds involved in tissue repair.

The destructive process and subsequent attachment loss progress apically. Tissue destruction is characterized by episodic periods of inactivity, which are probably linked with the reactivation of host defense mechanisms.

Attachment loss progressively pushes gingival sulcus tissues farther away from the offending bacterial biofilm. This may explain the discontinuous progression of periodontitis, which features alternating periods of reparative and destructive activities (Page et al 1997).

This process is comparable to a dynamic equilibrium, with periods of tissue destruction during which microbial virulence overcomes the host's defense capacity. In patients with advanced disease, the frequency of these active phases increases although the disease's progression phases are neither more aggressive nor longer in any given site. This implies that the host's defense mechanisms act locally to attempt to reestablish an equilibrium. Deep pockets are at a greater risk for high pathologic activity.

Histologic Alterations and Tissue Destruction

Toxins and enzymes produced by pathogenic anaerobic bacteria induce damage in periodontal tissues and initiate inflammatory processes. These enzymes can destroy extracellular matrix constituents such as collagen and damage the cell membranes of host cells. Microbial surface proteins also induce an immune response and local inflammation (Darveau et al 1997). Once inflammatory and immune responses are initiated, a host of molecules (including proteases, cytokines, prostanoids) is released by leukocytes, fibroblasts, or structural tissue cells. These proteases lead to a disorganization of the extracellular matrix by cleaving collagen molecules. This creates gaps into which leukocytes can further infiltrate periodontal tissue (Reynolds et al 1997). This destructive process is mostly regulated by host response. Gradually, periodontal tissues become more distended and more inflamed.

In periodontal disease, the connective attachment structures are destroyed, and epithelial cells proliferate and migrate apically along the root surface. The periodontal pocket deepens. Concomitantly, osteoclastic activity promotes bone destruction (Schwartz et al 1997). Subgingival plaque accumulates and microbial density increases, while host response becomes gradually more chronic and destructive.

Periodontitis and Systemic Disease

Periodontitis has been shown to represent a risk factor for atherosclerosis, pulmonary and cardiovascular disease (Beck et al, 1996), and premature delivery and low birth weight (Offenbacher et al 1996). The biofilm found at the surface of teeth is resistant; it reappears spontaneously after treatment and contains many gram-negative bacteria that continually discharge lipopolysaccharide vesicles. Bacteria and their by-products in the biofilm are in close proximity with periodontal connective tissues and can freely circulate inside the periodontal pocket.

By simply sweeping a curette through a periodontal pocket, one can collect up to 80 million culturable bacteria: in patients with advanced periodontitis, very highly loaded biofilms can be found. In an individual with 28 teeth, the total area of the biofilm has been estimated to be 72 cm^2, approximately the same surface area as the back of an adult hand. This represents an enormous burden of gram-negative bacteria! It is easy to imagine that this biofilm should directly affect vascular endothelial tissue and that it represents a risk for bacteremia both in clinical practice and during daily hygiene measures or mastication (Page et al 1997).

In Summary

- Periodontitis is an infection involving several bacterial species.
- Subgingival microbial populations organize into a structure called a *biofilm*; in so doing, subgingival flora assumes the properties of biofilms.
- Bacteria found in the biofilm initiate and maintain an immune-inflammatory response; this leads to destruction of connective tissue, periodontal ligament, and alveolar bone.
- Risk factors such as smoking or a genetic predisposition may alter the processes leading to tissue destruction and determine individual susceptibility to disease.
- Factors inherent to host response as well as environmental factors play an important role in the pathogenesis of periodontitis.
- Treatment is mostly based upon the reduction of subgingival and supragingival bacterial loads, along with the elimination or stabilization of modifiable risk factors.
- Scaling and root planing simultaneously reduce microbial load and enhance host immune response. This leads to clinical improvement and promotes the development of a new microbial balance.
- When active treatment leads to a significant reduction of inflammatory response, a reparative response is likely to occur.
- Suppression of certain bacterial species, in particular *P gingivalis* and *A actinomycetemcomitans*, usually involves additional antimicrobial chemotherapy.

- Periodontal surgery durably alters oral biofilm characteristics through reduction of probing depths and the disorganization of anaerobic microbiota (see section on the effects of surgical management on bacterial flora in chapter 4).
- Active therapy is concluded when the periodontal microbiota features a majority of gram-positive rods. This means the disease process has stabilized, and a new balance between host and flora has been established.
- Subsequent changes either in the flora or in host response may displace the equilibrium toward the renewal of pathologic processes and lead to further loss of attachment and gingival recession.

> The goal of periodontal treatment is to maintain healthy teeth in their positions on both arches. This goal can be reached when diagnosis and treatment planning are based on sound biologic data, ie, understanding of both infectious and inflammatory processes, in the light of modern clinical periodontal paradigms.

Diagnosis of Advanced Periodontitis

3

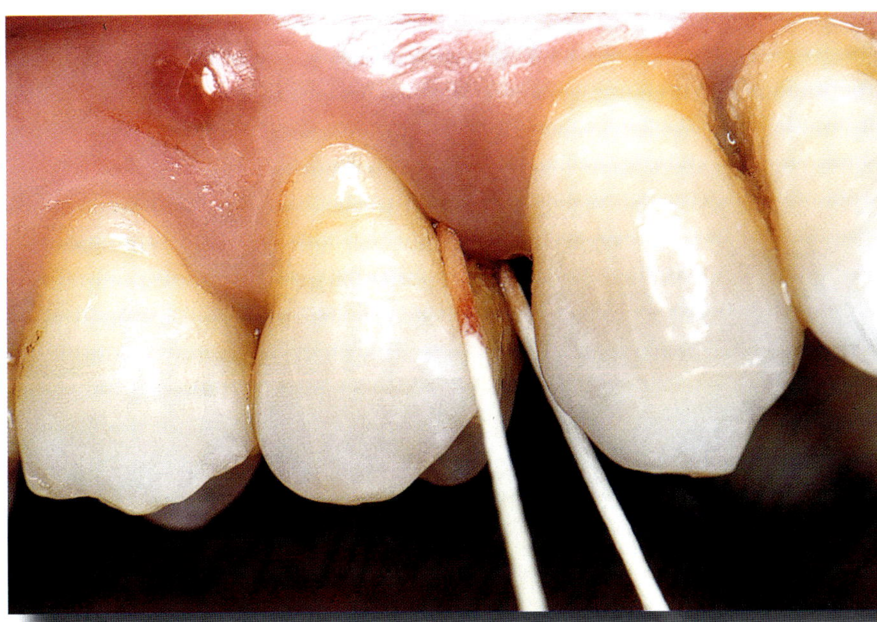

Classification

A new classification system for periodontal diseases was published in *Annals of Periodontology* in 1999. It was approved by the American Academy of Periodontology and was elaborated in accordance with the principles of evidence-based medicine.

This classification was intended to integrate epidemiologic, etiologic, and pathogenic data, and aimed at creating a rational classification system based on sound evidence rather than on clinical impressions. Only chronic and aggressive forms of periodontitis will be discussed in this book.

Gingivitis

Dental-plaque-induced gingival diseases

- Gingivitis associated with dental plaque only:
  - without other local contributing factors
  - with local contributing factors
- Gingival diseases modified by systemic factors
- Gingival diseases modified by medications
- Gingival diseases modified by malnutrition

Non-plaque-induced gingival lesions

Chronic periodontitis

Localized
Generalized

Aggressive periodontitis (Formerly juvenile, or precocious, or rapidly progressing periodontitis)

Localized
Generalized

Periodontitis as a manifestation of systemic diseases

Associated with hematological disorders (eg, leukemias)
Associated with genetic disorders (eg, Down syndrome, Papillon-Lefèvre syndrome)

Necrotizing periodontal diseases (eg, HIV infection)

Abscesses of the periodontium

Periodontitis associated with endodontic lesions

Developmental or acquired deformities and conditions

Localized and generalized forms of chronic periodontitis, while still referred to as *adult periodontitis*, are also observed in adolescents. However, there is little reason to associate these disease subtypes with a specific age category. Hence, a nonspecific terminology was preferred, and *chronic periodontitis* was deemed better-suited to describe the slow progression of the disease, though some patients may exhibit short periods of accelerated progression (Armitage 1999).

Clinical Signs and Symptoms of Periodontal Disease

An adequate evaluation of the clinical signs of periodontal disease is crucial not only for disease detection but also for recognition of disease type and severity. The collection of data leads to a diagnosis, orients treatment strategies, and allows for a prognosis to be made. This evaluation involves finding evidence of:

- Signs of inflammation
- Tissue damage

The usual parameters of destruction—attachment loss, pocket depth, bone loss, tooth mobility, and dental migrations—represent the historic aspects of disease progression. They help in appreciating severity but do not necessarily reflect the degree of pathologic activity. Pathologic activity is characterized by objective signs, such as the intensity of inflammation and presence of suppuration, and subjective signs, such as discomfort, tenderness, pain, and halitosis. However, the most significant sign is bleeding on probing. Again, periodontitis is known to progress discontinuously, and most of these clinical signs are present whether the disease is in an active or inactive phase. Taken together, these considerations emphasize the importance of developing better diagnostic and prognostic tests (Griffiths et al 1988). Microbiologic analysis seems a particularly powerful tool for proper evaluation of periodontal disease. This is discussed in the next chapter.

The readings recorded during periodontal probing are inaccurate if they are evaluated on inflamed tissue, because the probe can penetrate the inflamed connective tissue of the periodontal ligament. Correct scores are obtained only after reduction of inflammation.

The main treatment objective is to arrest periodontal destruction by eradicating inflammatory processes. Tissue repair, including attachment gain, reduction of pocket depth, mobility reduction, and bone repair, occurs once favorable biologic conditions have been established (Figs 3-1a and 3-1b). This naturally poses the problem of defining criteria necessary for periodontal stability in the four following situations:

- Healthy periodontium
- Pathologic periodontium (periodontitis)
- Treated periodontium
- Periodontium undergoing periodontal maintenance

Healthy periodontium

The most reliable criterion in assessing the stability of periodontal health is the absence of inflammation; this is generally demonstrated through the absence of bleeding on probing.

Pathologic periodontium

Criteria to evaluate periodontitis can be divided into four categories:

- Criteria used to assess the degree of inflammation
  - gingival appearance
  - presence of bleeding on probing
  - tooth mobility

- Criteria used to assess infectious etiology, as well as host susceptibility
  - presence of bacterial plaque
  - presence of pathogens
  - risk factors
- Criteria used to assess degree of severity
  - amount of bone destruction
  - amount of attachment loss
  - presence of deep periodontal pockets
  - tooth mobility
  - tooth displacement
- Criteria used to assess complexity
  - associated local factors
  - functional factors
  - esthetic factors

A treatment is considered successful when it changes the intensity of all features of disease. Some signs are totally reversible, others are not.

Treated periodontium

The purpose of elaborating evaluation criteria is for the assessment of treatment success. Treatment is considered successful when all reversible signs of disease have disappeared.

- Reduced plaque indices indicates reduced plaque loads and change in flora composition.
- Absence of bleeding on probing indicates reduced inflammation.
- Attachment gain indicates tissue response and initiation of reparative processes.
- Probing depth reduction indicates gingival retraction and attachment gain.

These criteria also help in assessing whether conditions suitable for periodontal stability have been achieved or not. These conditions are as follows:

- Host-bacteria balance has been reestablished.
- Conditions favorable to efficient plaque control have been attained.
- Risks factors are controlled.

Periodontium undergoing periodontal maintenance

The goal of supportive therapy is to prevent disease recurrence. Recurring inflammation is reversed by professional supportive therapy and does not systematically lead to a new period of destruction.

A site displaying repeated bleeding on probing more than likely presents attachment loss (Baderston et al 1985). The only reliable criterion for periodontal site stability is complete and sustained absence of bleeding on probing.

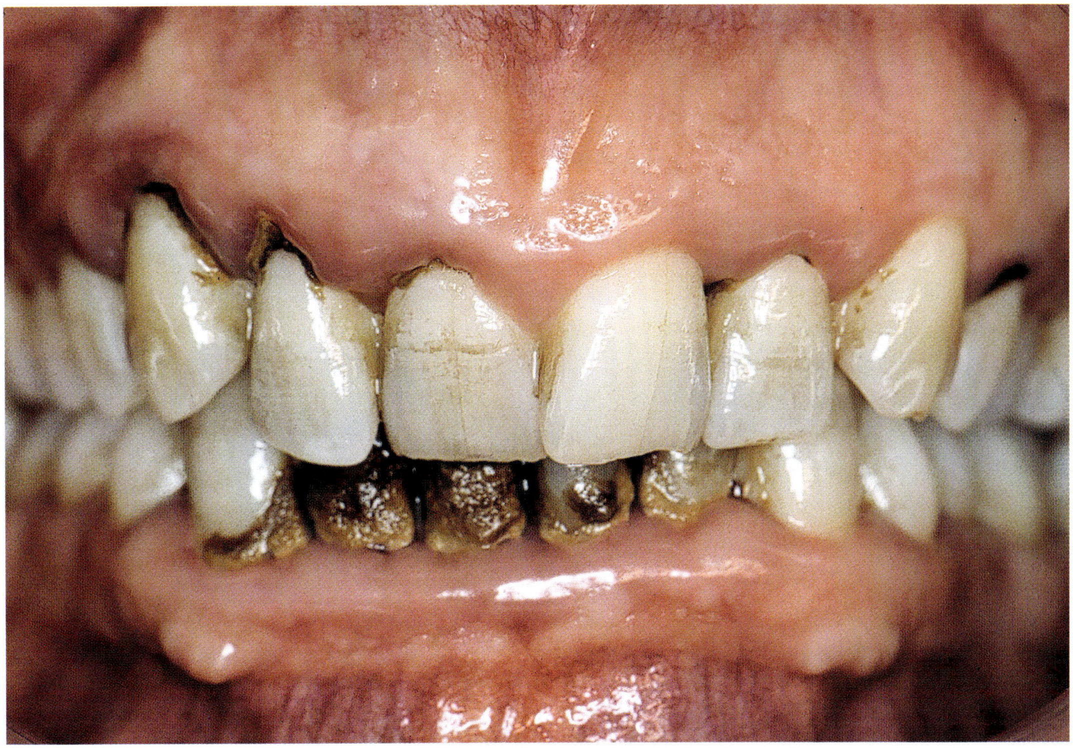

Fig 3-1a Periodontitis left untreated is characterized by a number of clinical and radiographic signs. These signs reflect the presence of inflammation (redness, swelling, bleeding), the level of severity (gingival recession, pockets, dental mobility and migrations, destruction), and infection (plaque deposits).

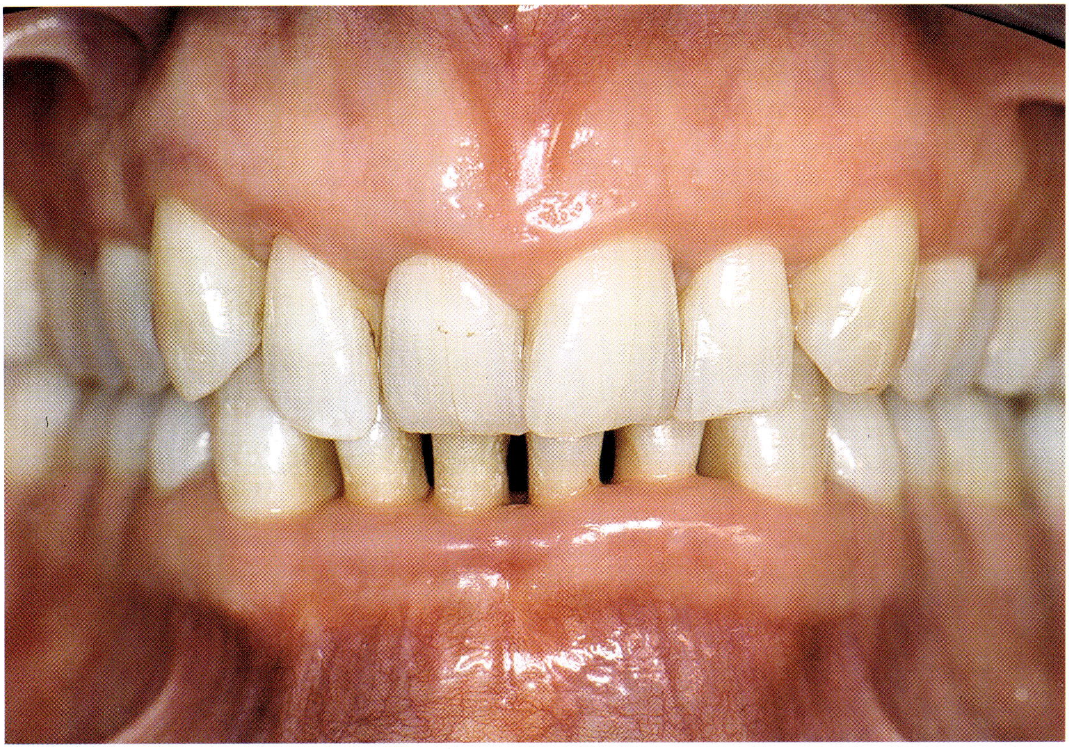

Fig 3-1b Clinical signs of inflammation are completely reversible; bleeding on probing disappears last. Successful management is characterized by progressive reversal of these clinical signs. Signs of destruction, on the other hand, are never totally reversible. At best, some amelioration can be observed (attachment gains, reduced migrations and mobility).

Microbiologic Diagnosis

The microbiologic treatment objective is achieved after exogenous pathogens—such as *Actinobacillus actinomycetemcomitans* or *Porphyromonas gingivalis* and bacterial species that belong to the red complex group—have been eradicated. A significant reduction in the commensal species counts is also sought.

P gingivalis, *Prevotella intermedia*, and *A actinomycetemcomitans* are the most important pathogenic species in aggressive, advanced periodontitis (Slots and Listgarten 1988). Their prevalence and relative numbers have been found to be higher in culture samples taken in active sites than in inactive sites. In addition, antibody titers are found to be significantly higher in the crevicular fluid and serum of subjects with periodontitis, compared with healthy subjects. Moreover, *P gingivalis* and *P intermedia* secrete powerful proteases, while *A actinomycetemcomitans* produces a variety of deleterious substances; these agents disrupt host defense mechanisms and thereby disintegrate some of the key constituents of periodontal tissue.

Persistence of these species in the periodontal pocket is a sign of persistent periodontal disease activity. Conversely, their disappearance is a good marker of treatment efficacy.

Microbiologic monitoring represents a crucial aspect in pursuing clinical success. Monitoring is performed at two levels: quantitative, the assessment of plaque indices; and qualitative, the determination of flora composition and screening for pathogenic species.

The clinical criteria that validate effective control of infectious processes are the following:

- Effective plaque control
- Renewed gingival health
- Absence or limited number of sites that bleed on probing
- Reduction of periodontal probing depths
- Attachment gain

These different clinical parameters are the consequence of tissue changes in response to microbiologic modifications, although they do not indicate the exact nature of these changes.

Clinicians now have the possibility of determining the nature and composition of the periodontal microbiota. This new clinical investigation has become an important, sometimes unavoidable, tool in establishing a diagnosis, selecting a treatment strategy, evaluating treatment efficacy, or in managing recurrent disease. As a general rule, microbiologic investigations are performed once satisfactory plaque control has been obtained, and occasionally after initial therapy (Figs 3-2 to 3-6).

Indications for microbial analyses

- Patients presenting with aggressive periodontitis.
- Patients who respond poorly to local treatment.
- Clinical situations involving a high risk for disease recurrence; microbiologic testing is all the more indicated when, in addition, treatment planning involves extensive surgical rehabilitation procedures, such as bone grafts, guided tissue regeneration, or extensive prosthetic treatment with or without further placement of dental implants.
- Younger patients presenting predisposing risk factors for periodontitis (family history of aggressive periodontitis, positive results of genetic screening tests)

- Young patients presenting with gingivitis or those scheduled to undergo orthodontic treatment.
- When attachment loss occurs in localized sites during periodontal maintenance.

Two very simple bacterial testing techniques are available: Bacterial sampling intended for cultural analysis and bacterial sampling intended for species-specific DNA-probes and polymerase chain reaction assays.

If the sample (see Fig 3-2) is intended for cultural analysis, the flask contains transportation liquid. This must be kept refrigerated until it is sent to the lab. Results are returned 4 to 5 weeks afterward.

If the sample is to be screened through molecular genetic techniques involving identification of bacterial DNA strands, the paper points are placed directly into the flask, without transportation liquid. The flask does not need to be refrigerated. Results are available after about 2 weeks.

Advantages of cultural analysis

- Precise quantitative (percentage) data are obtained.
- Antimicrobial sensitivity testing can be performed as indicated.
- Screening is possible for atypical microorganisms, including yeasts and enteric bacteria

Advantages of DNA probe assays

- There is no time limitation in expediting the sample to lab.
- Samples can be retrieved easily; transportation is simple.
- Results are returned in a short time.
- Screening for *Treponema denticola* (red complex spirochete) can be performed.

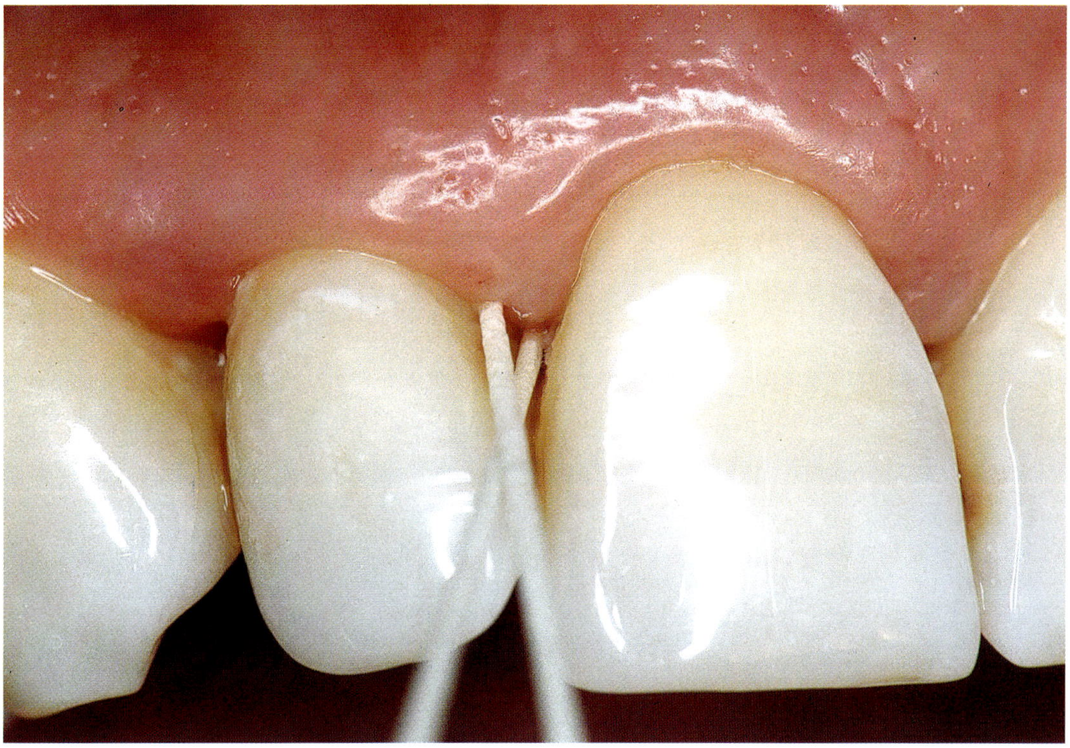

Fig 3-2 Supragingival plaque deposits are eliminated, and the sampling site is air dried. Four different sites were selected for analysis; all were characterized by the presence of pockets with probing depths exceeding 6 mm, bleeding on probing, and suppuration. A sterile paper point is inserted to the base of the given pocket for 10 seconds. The paper point is then placed in the transport vial. The procedure is repeated with a second paper point. Overall, eight paper points are used, two for each site.

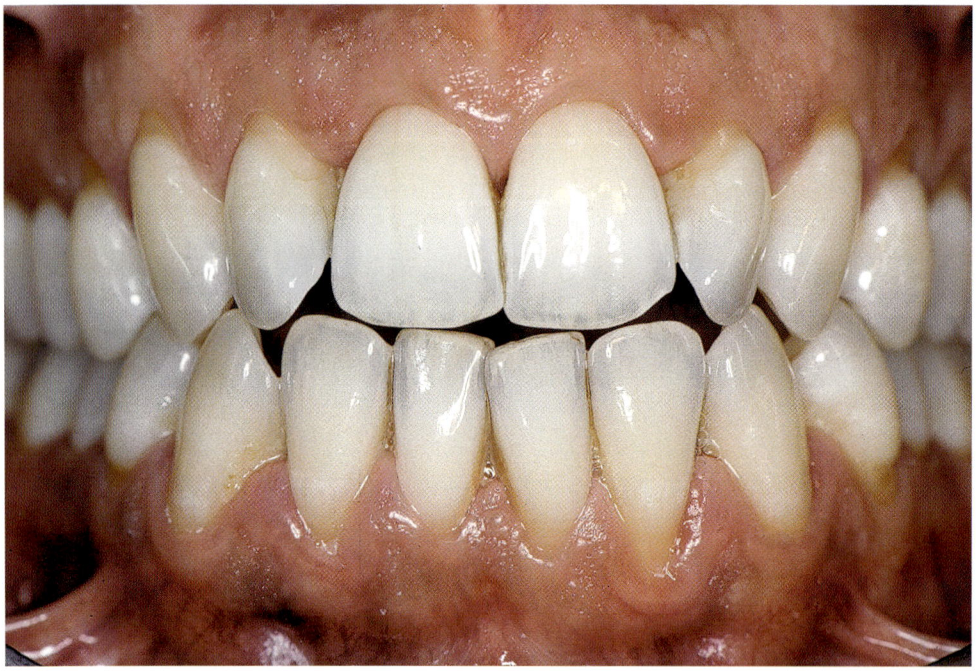

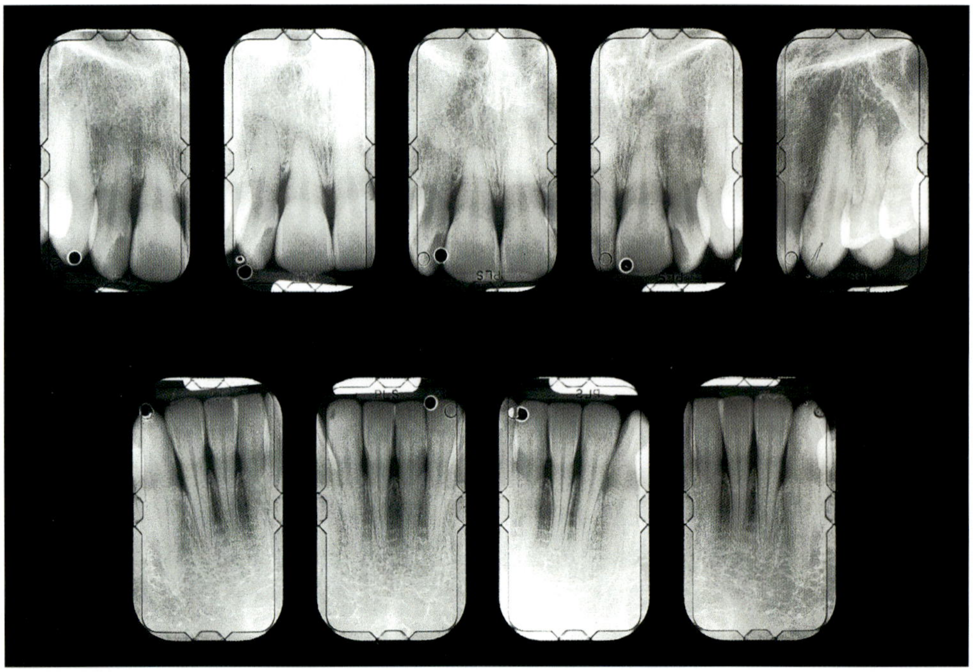

Figs 3-3a and 3-3b Female patient, 35 years old: smokes 20 cigarettes a day; otherwise healthy; brushes twice a day. Clinical signs of inflammation are discrete. Bone destruction is relatively severe (two-thirds of root height of maxillary right central incisor) and unevenly distributed. Culture analysis discloses presence of *Streptococcus mitis* (5.88%) and *Fusobacterium nucleatum* (22.22%) but no exogenous pathogenic species.

Diagnosis: Chronic periodontitis with commensal infection. How can the degree of severity be accounted for? Risk factors include tobacco use and stress. There may be a genetic predisposition that amplifies these risks.

Treatment strategy: Plaque control instructions + 3 toothbrushings per day + local treatment (scaling and root planing) + chlorhexidine + reduction or suppression of tobacco use. On the condition that tobacco reduction is significant, surgery will be performed for pockets with probing depths exceeding 4 mm. Periodontal maintenance.

Prognosis: Good, if the tobacco-related risk factor is eliminated. If the periodontal susceptibility test is positive, maintenance care should be intensified. If exacerbation of disease occurs, a new culture analysis should be performed.

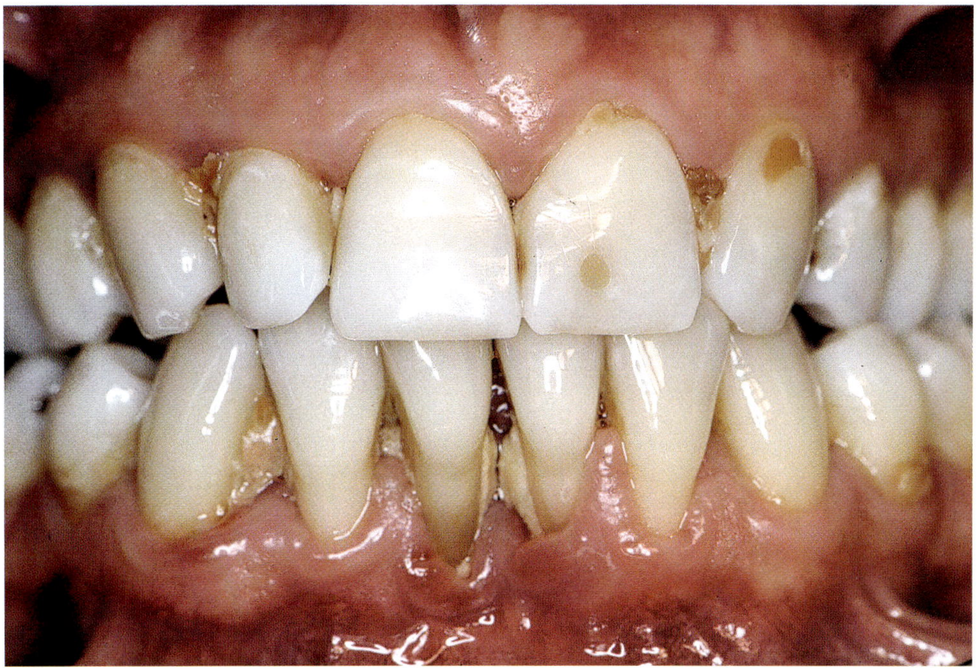

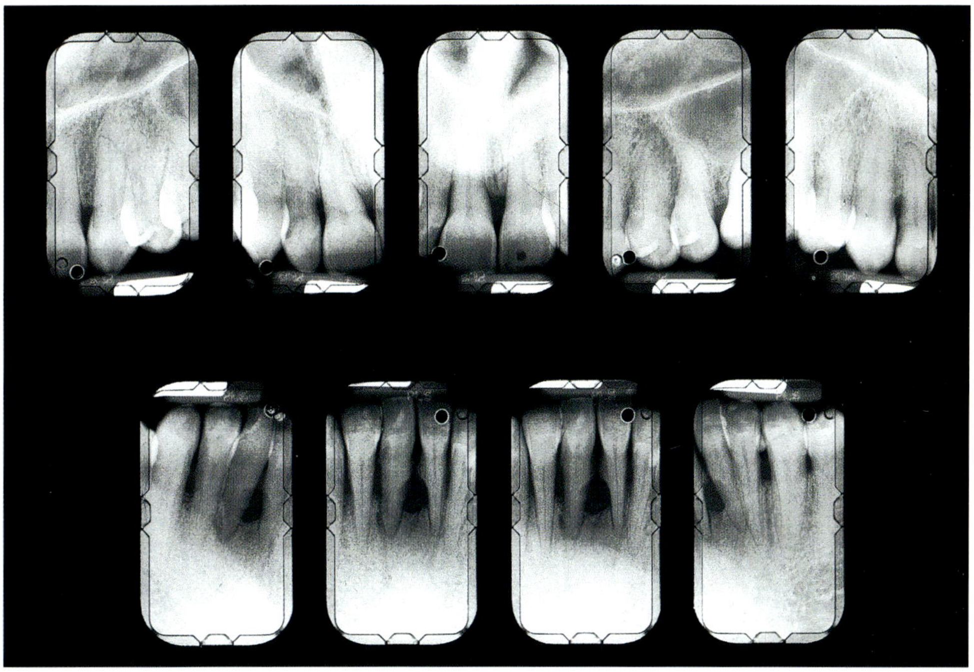

Figs 3-4a and 3-4b Female patient, 36 years old: smokes three cigarettes a day; reports history of rhinopharyngitis and family history of periodontal disease; brushes once daily. Clinical signs of inflammation are discrete and are more noticeable around mandibular incisors. Significant halitosis. Bone destruction is severe around mandibular incisors (Class III mobility and higher) and is more irregular in other areas. Four molars were already lost as a consequence of periodontal disease. Microbial analysis discloses *A actinomycetemcomitans* (1.61%), *P gingivalis* (14.00%), *Tannerella forsythensis* (12.50%), and *F nucleatum* (8.93%).

Diagnosis: Aggressive periodontitis with true periodontal infection by exogenous periodontal pathogenic species. How can the degree of severity be accounted for? Risk factors include a highly virulent pathogenic flora, probable predisposition, presence of functional factors, and occlusal dysfunction secondary to the loss of first molars.

Treatment strategy: Plaque control + 3 toothbrushings per day + local treatment (scaling and root planing) + antimicrobial therapy (amoxicillin 500 tid + metronidazole 500 mg tid) for 7 days + chlorhexidine + surgery in areas with deep pockets + functional rehabilitation and splinting of mandibular incisors. Periodontal maintenance.

Prognosis: Good, if pathogenic species are eliminated. Prognosis is reserved for mandibular incisors.

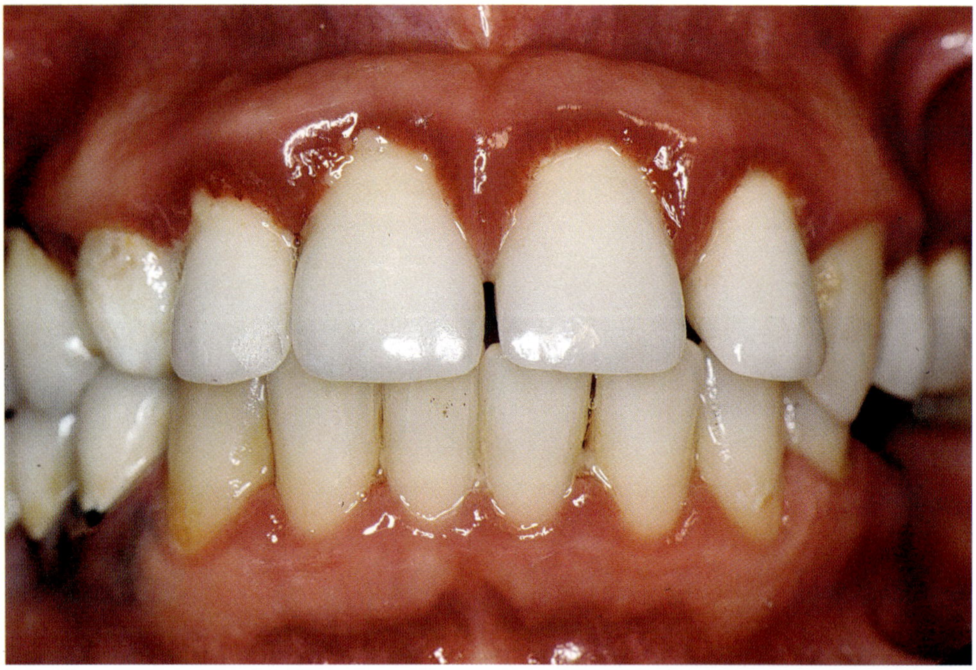

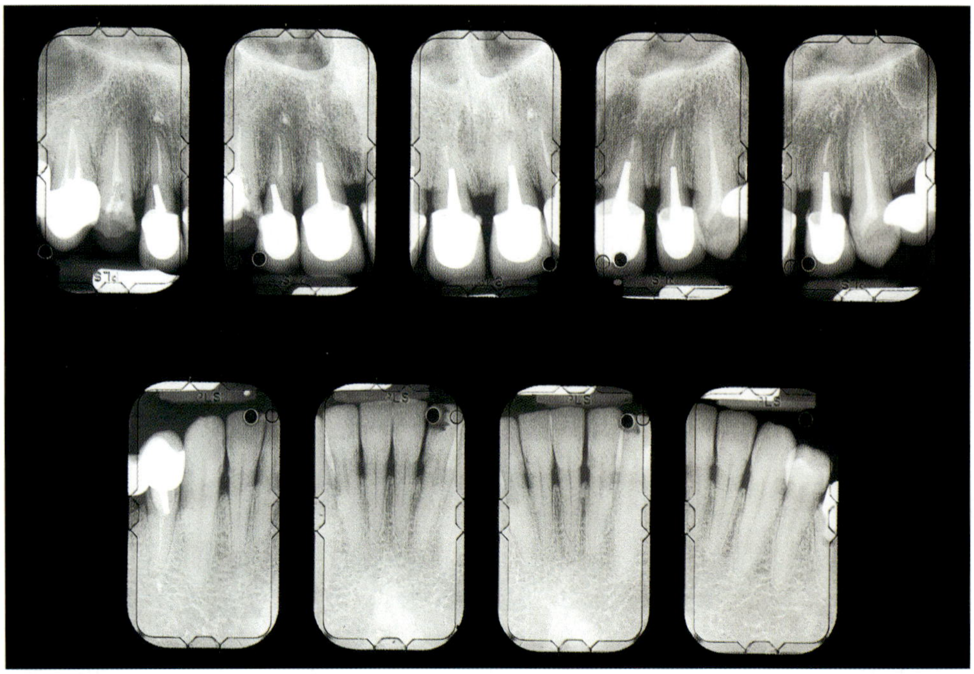

Figs 3-5a and 3-5b Female patient, 40 years old: nonsmoker; frequent labial herpetic lesions; fatigue; brushes once a day. Clinical signs of inflammation are important, especially around maxillary incisors. Significant halitosis. Bone destruction is marginal. DNA probing detects *A actinomycetemcomitans*, *P gingivalis*, *T forsythensis*, *T denticola*, and *F nucleatum*.
Diagnosis: Chronic periodontitis featuring dual infection by commensal species and periodontopathic exogenous species (red complex and *A actinomycetemcomitans*). Risk factors include extremely aggressive pathogenic flora, plaque index, and local factors (ie, unadapted prosthetic restorations). How can low degree of severity be accounted for? Very high patient resistance.
Treatment strategy: Plaque control + 2 toothbrushings per day + local treatment (scaling and root planing and provisional prosthetic restorations) + antimicrobial therapy (amoxicillin 500 tid + metronidazole 500 mg tid) for 7 days + preprosthetic surgery + chlorhexidine (0.12%). New fixed prosthetic restorations. Periodontal maintenance.
Prognosis: Very good.

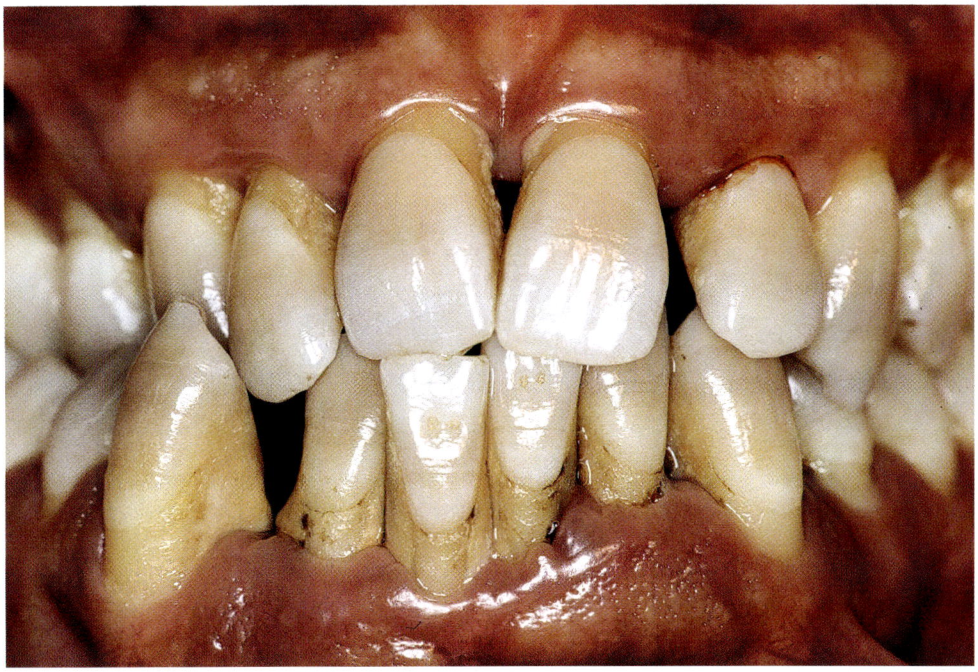

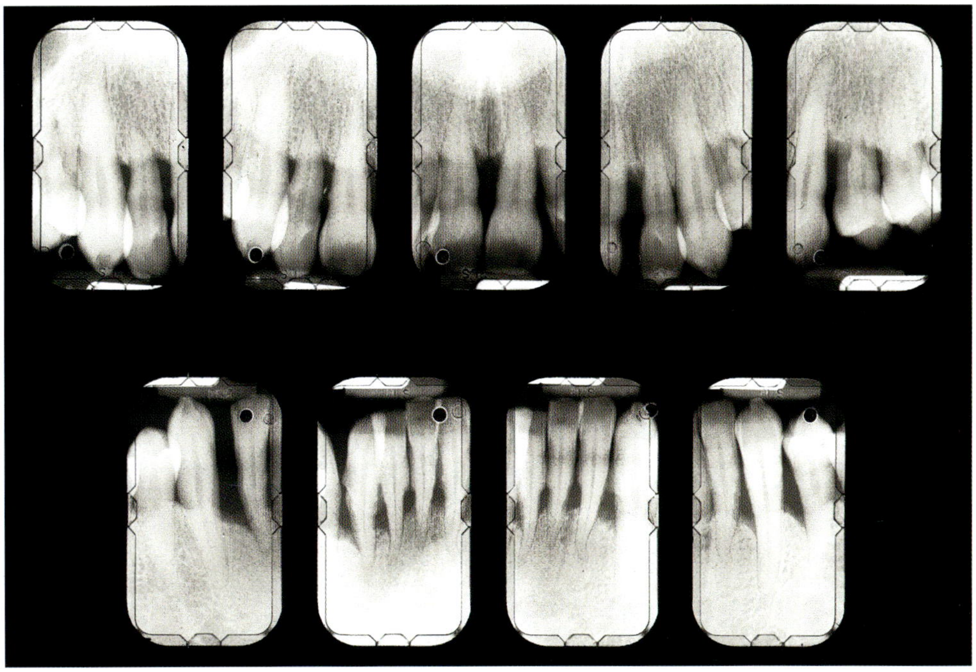

Figs 3-6a and 3-6b Male patient, 33 years old: quit smoking (10 cigarettes a day) 6 years ago; family history of periodontal disease; brushes once daily. There are important inflammatory signs, especially around mandibular incisors. Significant halitosis. Advanced, generalized bone destruction (Class III mobility and higher). Bacterial culture discloses *P gingivalis* (6.43%), *P intermedia* (11.90%), *T forsythensis* (7.14%), *Peptostreptococcus micros* (2.38%), and *F nucleatum* (2.38%).
Diagnosis: Aggressive periodontitis involving dual infection by commensal (*P intermedia*, *P micros*, and *F nucleatum*) and exogenous periodontopathic species (*P gingivalis* and *T forsythensis*). How can degree of severity be accounted for? Risk factors include pathogenic flora, probable predisposition, functional factor (primary occlusal factor), and prior tobacco use.
Treatment strategy: Plaque control + 3 toothbrushings per day + local treatment (scaling and root planing) + antimicrobial therapy (amoxicillin 500 mg tid + metronidazole 500 mg tid) for 7 days + surgery in areas with deep pockets + chlorhexidine (0.12%) + orthodontic treatment + splinting of anterior teeth + possible placement of dental implants to restore mandibular incisors. Periodontal maintenance.
Prognosis: Good, on the condition that pathogenic bacteria are eradicated. Prognosis is poor for mandibular incisors.

Microbiology of healthy and pathologic periodontal tissue

Unfortunately, there are no specific bacterial markers for periodontal health or for the different periodontal disease subcategories. However, frequent associations do exist between specific bacterial complexes and the different conditions of normal and pathologic periodontal tissue (Listgarten 1994).

Periodontal health	*Streptococcus sanguis* *Streptococcus mitis* *Veillonella parvula* *Actinomyces naeslundii* *Actinomyces viscosus* *Rothia dentocariosa*
Gingivitis	Species from *Actinomyces* genus Species from *Streptococcus* genus Species from *Veillonella* genus Species from *Fusobacterium* genus Species from *Treponema* genus *Prevotella intermedia*
Chronic periodontitis	Species from *Treponema* genus *Prevotella intermedia* *Porphyromonas gingivalis* *Tannerella forsythensis* *Peptostreptococcus micros* *Campylobacter rectus* *Actinobacillus actinomycetemcomitans* *Eikenella corrodens* Species from *Fusobacterium* genus Species from *Selenomonas* genus Species from *Eubacterium* genus
Localized aggressive periodontitis (previously juvenile periodontitis)	*Actinobacillus actinomycetemcomitans* Other species
Aggressive periodontitis	*Actinobacillus actinomycetemcomitans* *Porphyromonas gingivalis* *Tannerella forsythensis* *Campylobacter rectus* *Eikenella corrodens*

Since 1994, evidence of a strong association between some spirochete species (for example, *Treponema denticola*) and periodontal destruction has been found.

"Refractory" periodontitis (not a separate category in new classification)	*Actinobacillus actinomycetemcomitans* *Porphyromonas gingivalis* *Prevotella intermedia* *Tannerella forsythensis* *Campylobacter rectus* *Peptostreptococcus micros* Enteric rods Species from *Candida* genus

Complexity Factors

In a given individual, severity of periodontal destruction is not expressed uniformly in all areas of dentition (Baelum et al 1988) (Fig 3-7a).

Occasionally, infection by virulent pathogens in a given location may lead to massive localized periodontal destruction (see Fig 4-1). However, bacterial pathogens are usually not the only causative agents of infection. Bacterial etiology is also associated with local factors, which are either functional or secondary to periodontitis. These factors are termed *destructive cofactors* or *complexity factors*. The most frequently encountered are the following:

- *Local plaque retention factors:* High plaque scores lead to the development of periodontal disease in 80% of cases.
- *Presence of pathogenic species:* High pathogen counts, for instance, of *A actinomycetemcomitans* and other species belonging to the red complex, persisting for extended periods promote attachment loss.
- *Occlusal trauma:* When inflammation is absent, onset of tooth mobility due to occlusal trauma is reversible; in the presence of inflammation (periodontitis), periodontal destruction is aggravated.
- *Hyperfunctions and parafunctional habits:* Consequences similar to those with occlusal trauma are seen.
- *Periodontal pockets:* These are a consequence of tissue destruction and attachment loss. They are potential reservoirs for pathogenic species and consequently represent local risk factors for disease aggravation, especially when the probing depth exceeds 5 mm.
- *Bony and interradicular lesions:* These are sequelae of bone destruction and attachment loss and are frequently associated with deep periodontal pockets.
- *Dental mobility:* This is a consequence of inflammation and tissue destruction and may interfere with adequate control of plaque buildup. Persistent, elevated mobility levels (such as Class III mobility) should be considered an aggravating factor.

From a therapeutic point of view, the first goal should obviously be infection control, or reduction of inflammation, which is the clinical expression of infection. However, additional complexity factors need to be identified before they can be corrected or eliminated (Fig 3-7b). Each patient is characterized by a specific response to periodontal infection, which is related to personal risk factors, specific local factors, and an individual response potential.

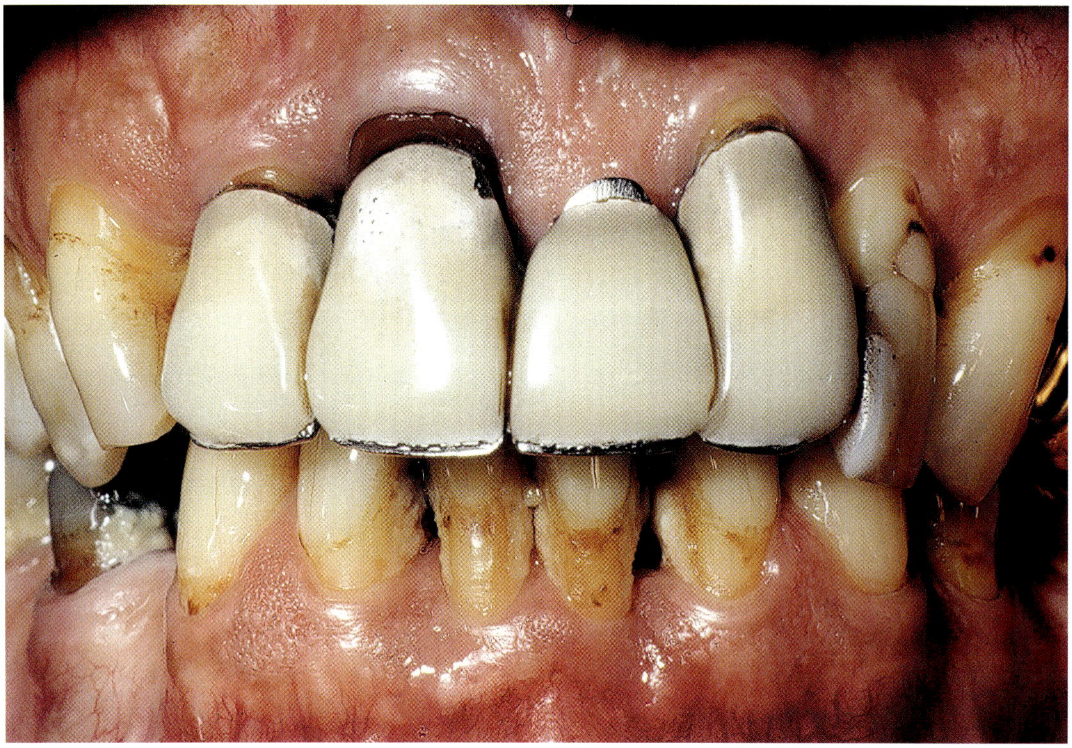

Fig 3-7a Usual signs of chronic periodontitis—gingival inflammation, modified gingival contour, and bacterial deposits—are exhibited.

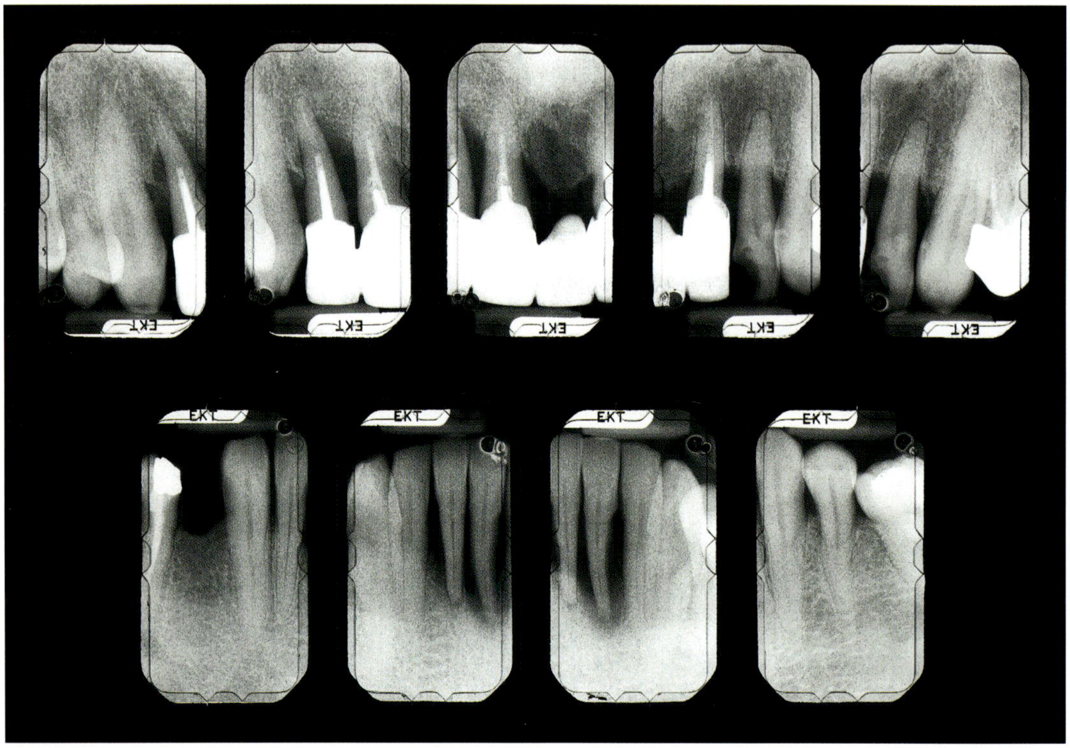

Fig 3-7b The radiographic signs of destruction illustrate the variability of periodontal destruction throughout the dentition; certain regions (mandibular canines and premolars) display virtually intact periodontal tissue, while others (maxillary and mandibular right incisors) present very high degrees of destruction. Local complicating factors have an influence on the destruction process and should be identified and either corrected or eliminated.

Infection Control in Periodontics

4

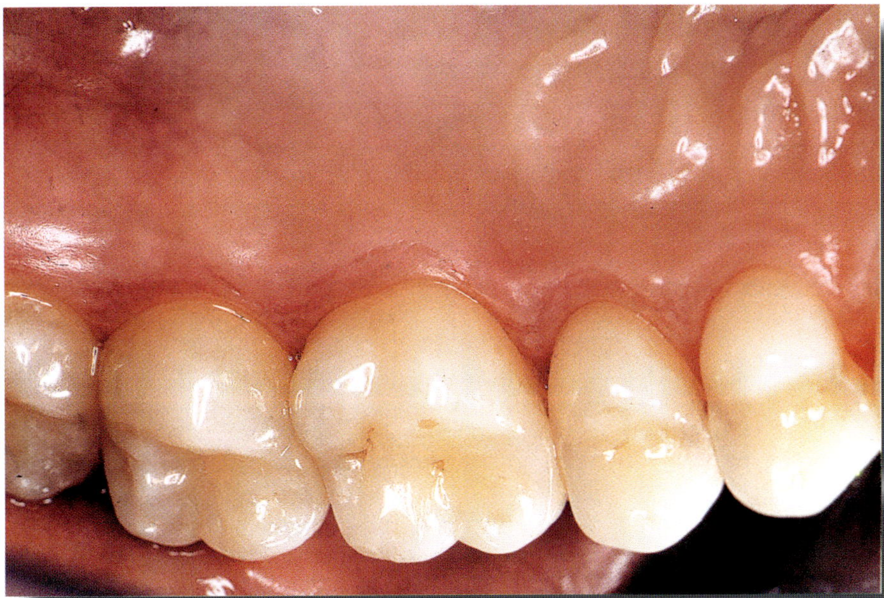

Criteria for Therapeutic Success

The rationale behind antimicrobial treatment in periodontal infections is easy to define; however, it proves more difficult to attain in practice. A new equilibrium between bacterial flora and periodontal tissues needs to be established, and any pathogenic agents present within the oral cavity must be eradicated. The difficulty in reaching these goals is mostly linked to the complex nature of bacterial reservoir sites and the difficulty in performing efficient hygiene procedures in these sites.

The periodontal pocket can be compared to an ecologic niche; this is further supported by the fact that edentulous patients and children present no pathogenic species. For an adult patient presenting with periodontal disease, the most significant risk factor for disease recurrence, among all measurable and bacteriologic clinical signs, is the persistence of periodontal pockets (Goodson 1994).

Conditions for clinical success are directly linked to effective infection control. These conditions are fulfilled once the attachment system has achieved stability, in the context of periodontal health. Variable results may be explained by:

- The presence of numerous etiologic factors, eg, high counts of different bacterial species involved in infection, species that are difficult to identify or culture, and sampling difficulties
- The diversity of clinical presentations: several disease subtypes lead to tissue destruction, and some may progress episodically
- The degree of severity linked to the presence of multiple risk factors, eg, systemic factors, difficulty in obtaining patient compliance, local factors such as those related to the condition of dentition

In treating advanced forms of periodontal disease, there are numerous conditions for success; these are directly correlated with the possibility of:

- Treating chronic and aggressive periodontitis globally
- Controlling all sites in a given patient
- Providing coordinated, multidisciplinary care designed to treat any dental involvement that may compromise periodontal health
- Knowing to what extent a tooth may be preserved when periodontal tissue is severely compromised.

Both esthetic and functional factors must be taken into account when managing advanced forms of severe periodontal disease where dental displacements, migrations, and edentulous areas are present. Prosthetic treatment options should be designed to allow optimal periodontal preservation and to facilitate periodontal maintenance.

Periodontal treatment per se is part of a more complex treatment strategy. Higher complexity levels are encountered when treatment success depends on nonperiodontal parameters; these include endodontic or orthodontic treatment procedures, splinting, provisional prosthetic constructions, implants, and other functional rehabilitation procedures.

Management of complex cases involves devising efficient modalities for treatment provisionalization. This is a difficult task and requires a lot of skill: an ill-fitted provisional crown may represent a local factor for treatment failure, and absence of a posterior occlusion is detrimental to treatment of periodontally compromised anterior teeth. Conditions for treatment success take into account all aspects of global treatment, while simultaneously ensuring stable control of infection.

Therapeutic procedures aiming at global treatment can be grouped into two categories:

- The first category includes the treatment procedures aiming at control of periodontal infection and reduction of bacterial load. The etiologic agent is eliminated or reduced until periodontal flora containing species compatible with periodontal health replaces pathogenic flora for a prolonged time. This is the first phase of periodontal management.
- The second category includes the treatment procedures aiming at repairing or restoring damaged dental and periodontal structures, thereby achieving functional restoration. This second phase cannot be initiated until the first phase has been successfully achieved. It will be described in the following chapters through clinical cases (see specifically the section on high-risk sites in chapter 6).

Periodontal microbiologic conditions can be modified in four different ways: through efficient plaque control, root scaling and planing, antimicrobial therapy (essentially antibiotic therapy), and surgery. At first, these four approaches seem easy to carry out; however, successful management of advanced periodontitis remains a difficult task because the efficacy of each of these methods is variable. Satisfactory results are achieved through a judicious combination of these four approaches.

Effects of Bacterial Plaque Control

The development of supragingival plaque precedes that of subgingival plaque; growth of the latter gradually selects pathogenic, anaerobic species, which exert toxic effects on periodontal tissue. Therefore, efficient plaque control measures should be established before any mechanical treatment is undertaken. Studies have shown that in patients with poor plaque control, there is a poor response to periodontal treatment (Nyman et al 1975); on the other hand, patients with chronic periodontitis who maintain good levels of plaque control are able to maintain satisfactory periodontal health over a 5-year period (Lindhe and Nyman 1975).

No invasive treatment should be initiated before significant improvement of plaque control.

Meticulous elimination of supragingival plaque, that is, reduction of plaque to indices below 20%, leads to significant alteration of the quantity and composition of subgingival bacterial flora (Dahlen et al 1992). Improvement of oral hygiene reduces bacterial load in deep pockets as well as in sites with lower probing scores, such as those found in gingivitis or untreated moderate periodontitis.

Growth of subgingival plaque can be reduced or arrested by toothbrushing and flossing. By limiting the accumulation of supragingival plaque, it is possible to interfere with the formation and maturation of pathogenic microbiota. Efficient supragingival plaque control deprives the subgingival environment of nutrients necessary to its growth. Also, supragingival plaque control reduces the intensity of gingival inflammatory response: inflammatory exudates, which represent an important source of nutrients for bacterial populations, are produced in smaller quantities (Listgarten 1999). In addition, adequate plaque control often means the patient is highly motivated and complies with recommendations given by the periodontist or dental hygienist. Individual hygiene is associated with regular professional periodontal maintenance, at a frequency determined according to the patient's personal risk factors.

Individual plaque control represents a first and crucial step in managing severe periodontal disease. Positive effects can be assessed through tissue response (reduced inflammatory signs) and through microbiologic change (a decrease in global bacterial load and in pathogen counts). Plaque control allows for maximum preservation of tissue and helps establish conditions favorable to microbiologic transformation.

Assessment of plaque control:
- Evaluation of plaque indices
- Evaluation of bleeding indices

Constant evaluation of plaque indices implies that the patient should brush after each meal. It is unacceptable for a patient to show up at an appointment without having brushed previously.

Effects of Scaling and Root Planing

Mechanical treatment consists of treating root surfaces manually with curettes or with ultrasonic scalers in order to eliminate the bacterial biofilm, endotoxins, calculus, and local factors contributing to plaque retention. Mechanical treatment includes supragingival scaling, subgingival scaling, and root planing. The overall objective of this aspect of treatment is to render root surfaces biologically compatible with the formation of a healthy new attachment apparatus.

Cementum elimination

Should all of the root's cementum tissue be eliminated? The biofilm is found at the surface of cementum tissue. Some toxins and bacteria are able to infiltrate the more superficial cementum strata, which consequently become unfit for the formation of a new attachment. The objective of scaling and root planing is to disorganize these bacterial niches and polish root surfaces while preserving a maximum amount of uninfected cementum (Figs 4-1a to 4-1c). This is a difficult task for several reasons:

- Cementum tissue width is reduced, and it is easily eliminated in just a few curette strikes.
- Complete absence of cementum prohibits the formation of new attachment tissue.
- Exposure of root dentin and dentinal tubules, especially when this occurs brutally, may cause root hypersensitivity and subsequent patient discomfort (Nyman et al 1988).

Calculus elimination and attachment gain

In terms of efficacy, there is no difference between manual instrumentation and ultrasound devices. However, manual scaling is 20% to 50% more time-consuming. Best results are obtained when both methods are combined (Sherman et al 1990).

- In small pockets with probing depths less than 4 mm, it has been estimated that up to 86% of calculus can be eliminated without resorting to surgical methods.
- In medium-depth pockets with probing depths ranging between 4 and 6 mm, up to 43% of calculus can be removed manually, compared with 76% surgically. Pocket depth reduction is more significant after surgical intervention.

- In deep pockets featuring probing depths exceeding 6 mm, 32% of calculus can be removed manually, compared with 50% surgically. Pocket depth reduction and attachment gain are more important after surgical treatment. Recurrence is more frequent when initial treatment consists of root scaling and planing only, compared with root scaling/planing in conjunction with periodontal surgery (Ramfjord et al 1987; Becker et al 1988).
- In invaded furcations, elimination of calculus is always somewhat random, as are clinical attachment gains, compared with gains obtained for monoradicular teeth (Loos et al 1988). Surgical access to the site improves calculus elimination, with a removal rate no higher than 68%, regardless of the clinician's experience. This efficacy rate decreases as periodontal pocket depth increases (Fleischer et al 1989).

After 24 months, attachment loss increases in 25% of molar-furcation cases, compared with 10% for molars with flat-surface sites (Loos et al 1989). In another study, similar clinical improvements were found among nonsmokers and ex-smokers but not among subjects who smoked at the time of study (Haffajee et al 1997).

Bleeding indices

Bleeding indices improve in sites where pocket depth is equal to or less than 4 mm, but they remain high in deeper pockets. In furcations, initial values return 24 months after root scaling and planing (Loos et al 1989).

Bacterial flora

Combined root scaling and planing allow for a relative increase in the total numbers of beneficial bacteria and reduce bacterial loads and the amount of pathogenic species present in all sites, except in furcations where the bacterial load decrease is less significant (Loos et al 1988). *Porphyromonas gingivalis* is eliminated from most sites whereas *Actinobacillus actinomycetemcomitans* tends to persist in different sites (Renvert et al 1990).

Where probing depths exceed 6 mm, there is a significant decrease in the number of pathogens from the red complex (*P gingivalis*, *Treponema denticola*, *Tannerella forsythensis*) in nonsmokers. In smokers, on the contrary, there is an increase in bacterial population numbers. *P gingivalis* counts tend to decrease in all pocket subtypes. *T forsythensis* counts seem to decrease only in small pockets (Haffajee et al 1997).

Taken together, these elements illustrate the difficulty posed by deep lesions and furcations when they are treated nonsurgically. In these cases, it is necessary to resort to other treatment modalities.

Root scaling and planing treatment procedures are not sufficiently effective to eliminate red complex bacterial populations altogether. Neither do they suffice to remove all root calculus, particularly that found in deep pockets. Surgical management significantly improves clinical results obtained after root scaling and planing. However, the outcome is not as favorable in smokers as it is in nonsmokers. Potential for repair in severely compromised sites becomes apparent during the first series of scaling and root planing sessions, which, in the case of severe periodontal disease, are usually performed in four to six consecutive sessions. Treatment rationale therefore requires that scaling and root planing be initiated immediately after the patient has acquired satisfactory plaque control. To reduce tissue damage, local anesthesia is avoided as much as possible.

In deep pocket sites (probing depths exceeding 6 mm) clinical improvement can be significant, though only limited change occurs in the subgingival microbiota. When treating advanced forms of periodontitis with numerous deep pockets, ample time intervals should be worked into the treatment schedule to allow for a favorable tissue response. Persistence of pathogenic bacteria or biofilm fragments can represent an indication for antibiotic therapy because there is a strong risk for recurrence. In these cases, guidelines for treatment are the following:

- ***First phase:*** Plaque control plus mechanical treatment consisting of scaling and planing without local anesthesia plus postoperative assessment of attachment gains and potential for repair. The rationale behind root planing without anesthesia is to avoid any damage to the protagonists of reparative tissue response.
- ***Second phase:*** This additional treatment step includes administration of antibiotic therapy, preferably after microbiologic analysis, followed by repeated mechanical treatment (this time under local anesthesia) involving root planing and periodontal surgery. The goals of this second treatment phase are defined according to the outcome of the first treatment phase. Here again, the overall objective is to improve pathogen and bacterial biofilm elimination to better prevent recurrence. Whenever

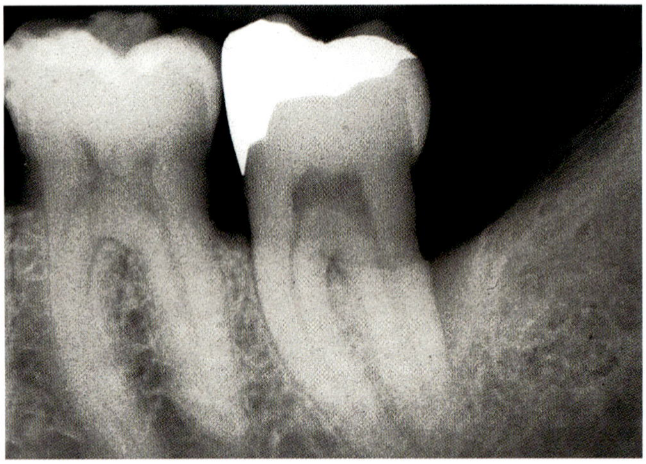

Fig 4-1a Deep bony lesion after several years of periodontal maintenance. Despite good plaque control, there is evidence of periodontopathic species colonization (*P gingivalis*, 30%; *T forsythensis*, 1%; *Peptostreptococcus micros*, 26%). Antibiotic therapy was initiated.

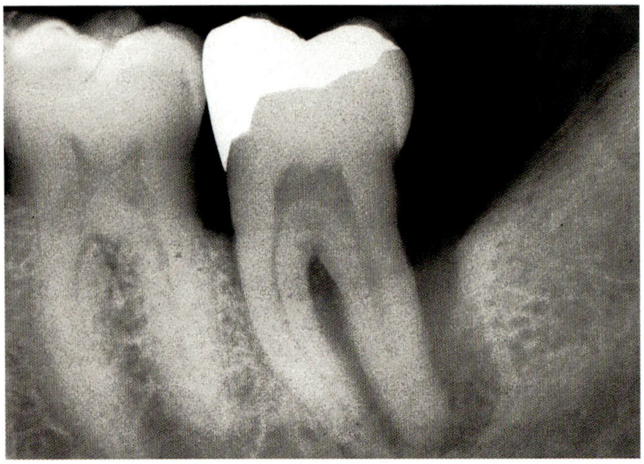

Fig 4-1b Acute infectious complication 6 months later.

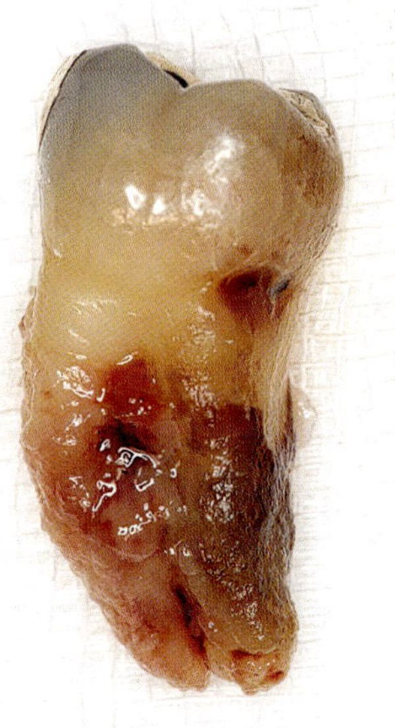

Fig 4-1c The tooth was extracted. Note the limited efficacy of scaling and root planing in biofilm elimination.

clinical improvement is deemed limited despite satisfactory plaque control, microbiologic analysis is probably warranted.

Evaluation of mechanical treatment outcome:
- Evaluation of bleeding on probing index
- Charting of probing depth
- Charting of attachment loss

It is reasonable to expect that for most pockets with probing depths less than 5 mm, bleeding on probing will cease and a decrease in probing depth will occur (gingival retraction and/or attachment gain).

Effects of Antibiotic Therapy

The goal of systemically administered antibiotic therapy is to eliminate pathogenic species and, subsequently, to select the development of microbiota compatible with periodontal health. Occasionally, when treating acute infection, early antibiotic therapy is indicated to reduce infection before initiating mechanical treatment. Regeneration of connective attachment tissue cannot be expected while *P gingivalis* populations persist. As a general rule, antibiotic treatment improves the outcome of mechanical treatment and promotes host defense mechanisms by acting on subgingival pathogens that are resistant to mechanical treatment (Van Winkelhoff et al 1996). Several factors account for the difficulty in reaching this objective: the limited, specific activity spectra of antibiotic compounds, difficulty in reaching appropriate antibiotic concentrations in infected sites, and finally, the biofilm's characteristics. Many antibiotics have been used empirically. Currently, the most efficient compounds are known to be amoxicillin and metronidazole.

Effect of antibiotic therapy combined with scaling and root planing

The combination of amoxicillin (375 mg tid for 7 days) plus metronidazole (250 mg tid for 7 days) plus root scaling and planing leads to a better clinical and microbiologic outcome than scaling and root planing alone. Patients who test positive for *P gingivalis* respond particularly well to antibiotic treatment (Winkel et al 2001). This same combination eradicates *A actinomycetemcomitans* populations over an extended period (24 months) in patients whose periodontal disease is related to this species (Pavicic et al 1994). Comparative studies of treatments with amoxicillin (500 mg tid for 14 days) or with metronidazole (250 mg tid for 14 days) regimens, administered concomitantly with scaling and root planing, show that:

- Both antibiotics induce rapid reduction in the numbers of several species from the red complex (*T forsythensis, P gingivalis,* and *T denticola*).
- At day 360, a rebound effect occurs for populations from the red complex in patients treated with amoxicillin but not in patients treated with metronidazole.
- In both groups, bacteria counts from the orange complex decrease, but they increase again 90 days after the end of antibiotic therapy.
- Counts of compatible species belonging to the orange and yellow complexes tend to increase during antibiotic therapy and decrease afterward (Feres et al 2002).

  How can this rebound of red-complex species be accounted for, when treating with amoxicillin and scaling and root planing? Also, why does this rebound effect not occur after treatment with metronidazole and scaling and root planing?

Scaling and root planing procedures reduce pathogenic red-complex bacteria numbers in the periodontal pocket without eliminating them altogether. A new colonization may arise from residual pocket bacteria or biofilm fragments, though antibiotic therapy may have led to a significant reduction in tissue bacterial load. Amoxicillin is probably less efficient than metronidazole in reducing red-complex bacterial loads in periodontal pockets.

Taken together, these elements suggest that antibiotic therapy should not be initiated before a significant decrease in subgingival bacterial loads has been achieved.

Why did the pathogenic bacteria from the orange complex, whose numbers decreased in both groups, increase again?

These bacteria are mostly commensal; their ability to organize into a biofilm accounts for their poor response to antibiotic therapy. This justifies the association of mechanical scaling and planing therapy with antibiotic treatment in a second treatment phase.

Actinobacillus actinomycetemcomitans

This species can survive more than 20 years in untreated periodontal lesions. Host defense mechanisms as well as professional scaling and root planing are insufficient to eliminate these populations altogether. Periodontal surgery seems to induce a limited reduction in *A actinomycetemcomitans* counts. Tetracyclines eradicate *A actinomycetemcomitans* populations in juvenile forms of periodontitis, but they remain largely inefficient in other forms of periodontal disease (Slots and Ting 1999). A combination of amoxicillin and metronidazole (250 to 500 mg tid for 8 days) is now recommended for treatment of infections involving this bacterial species, especially if they are associated with multiple other pathogenic species with differing antimicrobial susceptibilities. This antibiotic combination may be associated with an increased risk for sensitization; however, an empirical prescription is associated with a higher risk for selecting resistant bacterial strains.

Pocket depth and attachment level

Treatment with amoxicillin and metronidazole, combined with scaling and root planing, leads to overall attachment gains and a significant decrease in pocket depths in patients with advanced or refractory forms of periodontitis (van Winkelhoff et al 1992). Also, therapy with either amoxicillin or metronidazole is associated with the following changes (Feres et al 2001):

- Little change in pockets with depths inferior to 4 mm
- Moderate though significant attachment gains for pocket depths ranging from 4 to 6 mm
- Significant attachment gains for pocket depths exceeding 6 mm

These results are seldom sufficient. In deep pockets, scaling and root planing are not sufficient to completely eliminate the biofilm; this increases the risk for recurrence, even though an important attachment gain may well have occurred. Additional mechanical treatment is warranted for further reduction in pocket depth, just as it is for the elimination of pathogenic bacterial populations. This has been confirmed in a recent study showing that treatment with metronidazole, administered concomitantly with a second phase of thorough scaling and root planing performed under local anesthesia, efficiently eliminates periodontal pathogenic bacteria, induces an increase in host response, and promotes significant attachment gain, compared with treatment with doxycycline or scaling and root planing used alone (Sigusch et al 2001).

Assessment of antibiotic treatment efficacy:
- Bleeding on probing scores
- Mobility assessment
- Assessment of attachment gains, pocket depth reduction, mobility reduction
- Radiographic evaluation (bone gain)

Treatment planning for infection control

When evaluating deep pockets containing pathogenic bacteria, the clinician needs to address several important questions: which is the best treatment protocol, what is the appropriate timing for antibiotic therapy, and which antibiotic should be used?

The data presented earlier suggest that after rapid reduction of pathogenic bacterial load through initial mechanical treatment, and while this bacterial load is at its lowest, additional local treatment should be initiated. This may involve a second phase of intensive scaling and root planing or periodontal surgery. These procedures prolong the beneficial effects of the initial treatment phase and promote periodontal stabilization (Figs 4-2a to 4-2d). This second phase is performed under local anesthesia, which is justified by the fact that tissue and microbiologic healing is already well under way (Figs 4-3a to 4-3f). Treatment protocol is as follows:

- ***First phase***
  - Oral hygiene instructions (Bass method)
  - Supra- and subgingival scaling, root planing, and polishing in three to five consecutive visits
  - Microbial monitoring
- ***Second phase***
  - Antibiotic therapy
  - Intensive root scaling in all quadrants, under local anesthesia in one or two close sessions, plus surgical dressing

Corrective or regenerative periodontal surgery procedures are not to be performed before infection is thoroughly controlled.

Treatment of periodontal infection represents an ecological dilemma. The problem is the elimination of pathogenic species without altogether eradicating beneficial species or those that are compatible with periodontal health (Socransky et al 1999). However, there is no clearly drawn line between beneficial bacterial populations and those associated with disease. Hence the most appropriate treatment modalities are those that take into account the subtle gradations that differentiate these bacterial groups and avoid inducing a microbiologic catastrophe. Clinical improvement is the prime criterion in selecting a treatment strategy. This means that proper control of both supra- and subgingival ecosystems should be achieved.

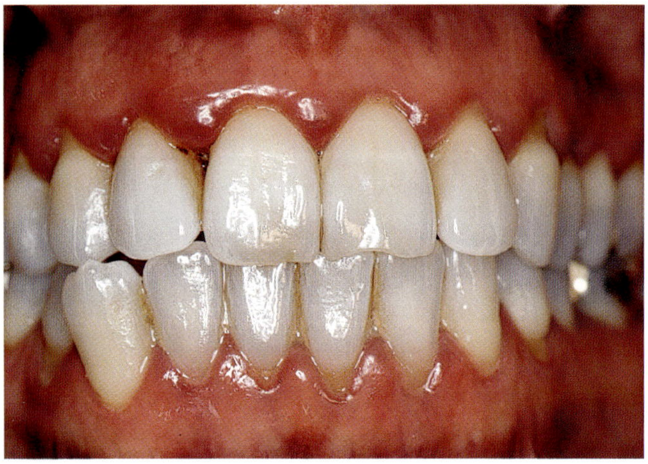

Fig 4-2a Periodontitis in a 38-year-old female patient. The patient never underwent tooth cleaning, and there is a significant amount of bacterial deposit. Despite the presence of significant inflammation, the working diagnosis was chronic periodontitis.

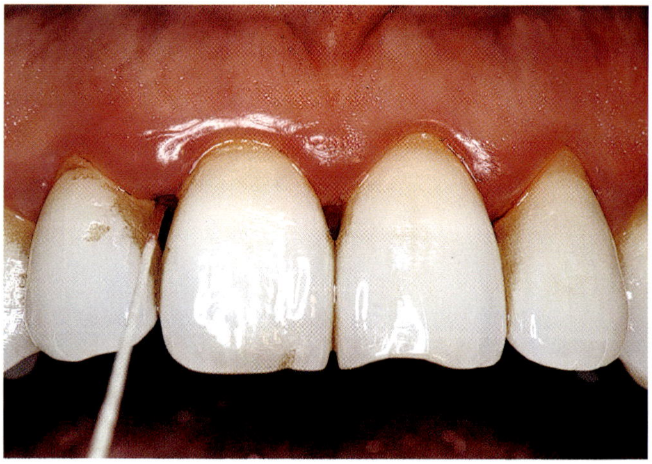

Fig 4-2b The outcome after four initial treatment sessions (root scaling and planing two times each) is very disappointing. Bacterial culture discloses the presence of pathogenic species from the red complex (*P gingivalis*, *T forsythensis*, *T denticola*).

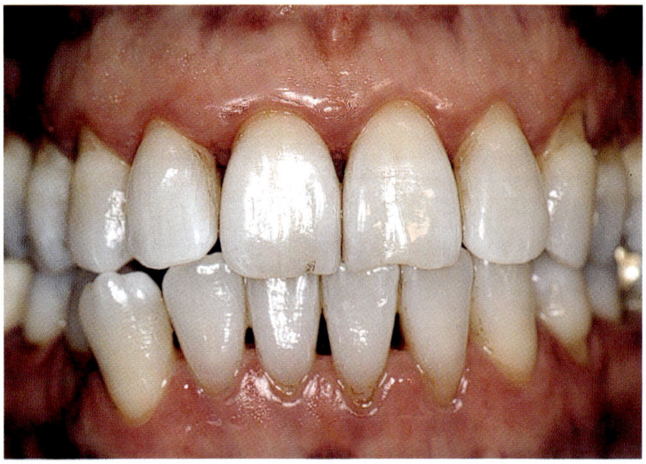

Fig 4-2c Two weeks after a 7-day course of antibiotic therapy (metronidazole 500 mg tid) with chlorhexidine-associated toothbrushing, gingival health has clearly improved.

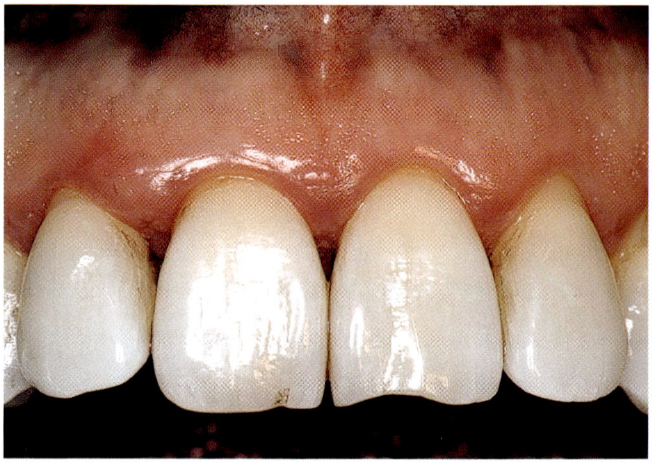

Fig 4-2d At this point additional treatment is necessary to improve root planing in several interproximal regions. Some residual plaque biofilm persists; its physical characteristics may account for antibiotic treatment failure and recurrence of inflammation. Biofilm elimination is optimized by use of local anesthesia.

Antibiotic therapy is not, in and of itself, sufficient treatment for periodontal disease, although it needs to be integrated into the general treatment strategy. Antibiotic therapy is initiated when infection signs persist despite reduction of bacterial load through local measures. It is often indicated for smokers.

When dealing with a virulent, complex flora (ie, *A actinomycetemcomitans* plus other pathogenic species), combined use of amoxicillin and metronidazole (250 to 500 mg tid for 8 days) is recommended. For periodontal flora featuring *P gingivalis* associated with commensal species, use of metronidazole alone is preferred.

Efficacy of antibiotic therapy is linked both to duration of the prescription (7 to 10 days) and to its appropriate timing in treatment. Coupling treatment with use of chlorhexidine or surgery is often advisable.

The broad spectrum of amoxicillin justifies that it should be chosen for first-line treatment.

Effects of Surgical Therapy on Bacterial Flora

Overall, nonsurgical treatment does not eliminate periodontal pathogens altogether, though a significant decrease in their numbers does occur. In contrast, pathogens are undetectable during a 1-year period following periodontal surgery (Widman flap procedure) (Rawlinson et al 1995). However, surgery does not completely eliminate *A actinomycetemcomitans* (Renvert et al 1990).

Effect of scaling and root planing

The effects of root planing and scaling alone were compared to those observed after root planing and scaling associated with osseous surgery performed during an apically repositioned flap surgery procedure (Levy et al 1999):

- Total bacterial load is significantly reduced after scaling and root planing.
- Surgery induces a significant decrease in bacterial counts from the orange complex.
- *P gingivalis* populations are completely eliminated from surgically treated sites.

In addition, sites treated with bone surgery present no probing depth exceeding 5 mm, and no pathogenic bacteria are found in these sites.

In contrast, patients treated without surgery feature many persistent pockets and high pathogenic species counts of *A actinomycetemcomitans*, *Prevotella intermedia*, *P micros*, and *P gingivalis,* as well as mobile rods (Nowzari et al 1996).

When bone craters are present, flap surgery involving bone recontouring is associated with greater pocket depth reductions and improvement of pathogen counts than is surgery involving an apically repositioned flap without bone recontouring. After bone surgery, *A actinomycetemcomitans* and *P gingivalis* are no longer detected. When bone surgery is not performed, there is an increase in *A actinomycetemcomitans* numbers, though *P gingivalis* counts remain stable (Tuan et al 2000).

Long-term outcome of surgical treatment compared with nonsurgical treatment

The short-term positive outcome of surgical management has been investigated. Similarly, long-term benefits have been shown to exist (Serino et al 2001).

Surgical treatment leads to better outcome than nonsurgical treatment for elimination of bacterial species belonging to the red complex and *A actinomycetemcomitans* and for reduction of deep pockets (probing depths exceeding 6 mm).

For patients undergoing maintenance therapy (three to four sessions per year), signs of disease progression are more frequent in patients who were treated nonsurgically. In the long term (13 years), there are fewer reports of recurrence in surgically treated patients and therefore fewer indications for further treatment.

Which surgical treatment should be selected?

A single treatment plan cannot be considered adequate for all clinical cases; similarly, a single surgical approach to periodontal disease cannot be proposed for treatment of all anatomic locations. The goals of periodontal surgery should be clearly defined, and surgical techniques must be tailored to individual cases.

Fig 4-3 Effect of surgical treatment.

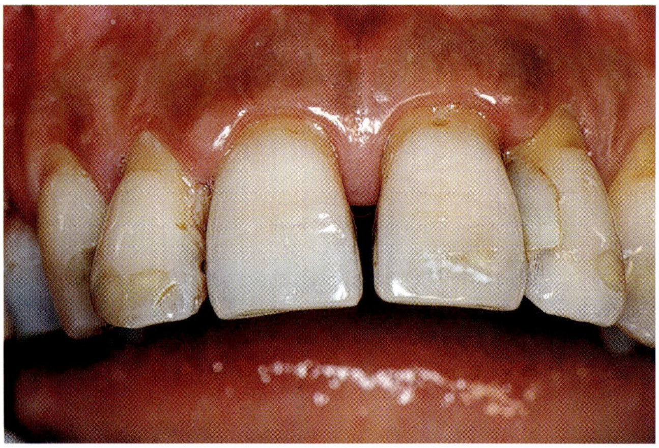

Fig 4-3a Aggressive periodontitis in a 28-year-old female smoker who is subject to stress and has a family history of periodontal disease. Few plaque or calculus deposits are present. Bacterial screening discloses no highly pathogenic species except *Eikenella corrodens*, which is resistant to most antibiotics and secretes osteolytic phosphatases.

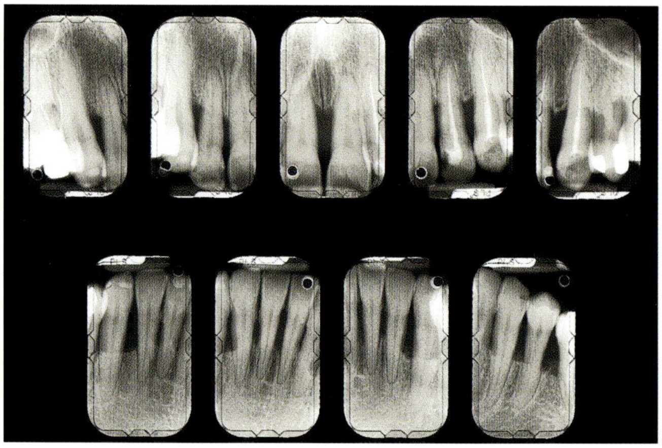

Fig 4-3b Destruction is severe, greater than 50%. Probing depths exceed 6 mm. Migrations and diastemata are of recent onset. Incisor mobility is Class II. Severity is related to host response.

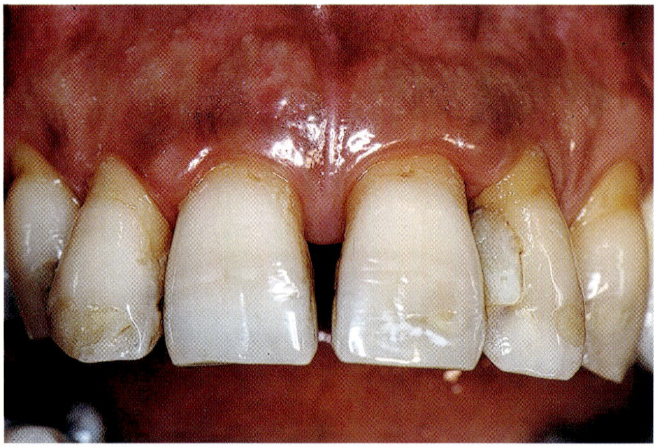

Fig 4-3c After initial therapy (scaling and two root planing sessions), clinical improvement is very limited. There is slight bleeding on probing (bleeding is always limited in smokers).

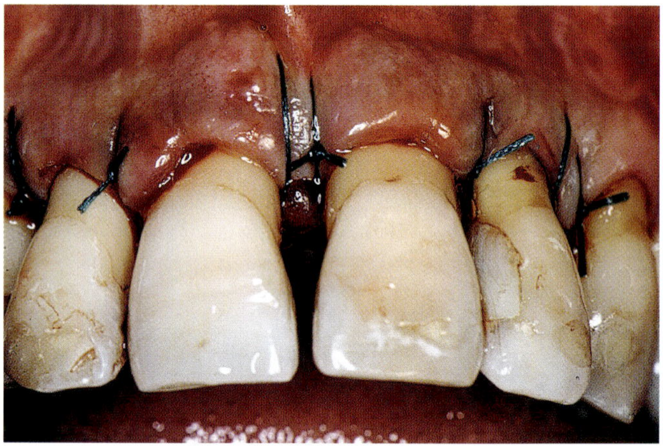

Fig 4-3d Periodontal flap surgery (pockets are deeper than 6 mm) is performed in conjunction with a 7-day course of amoxicillin (prophylaxis in a susceptible patient).

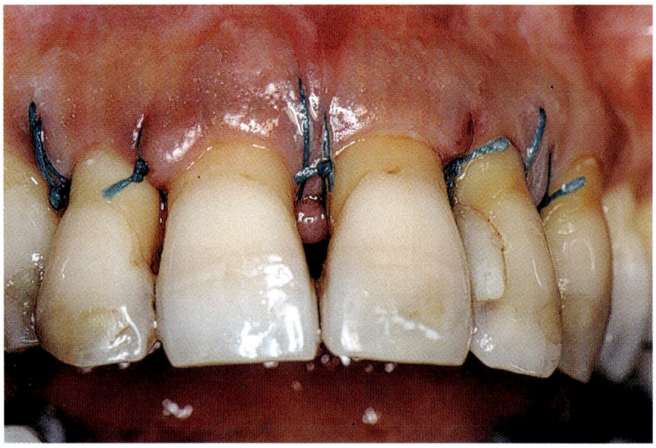

Fig 4-3e One week later, healing is normal and a significant reduction of mobility has occurred. This indicates an arrest in disease progression.

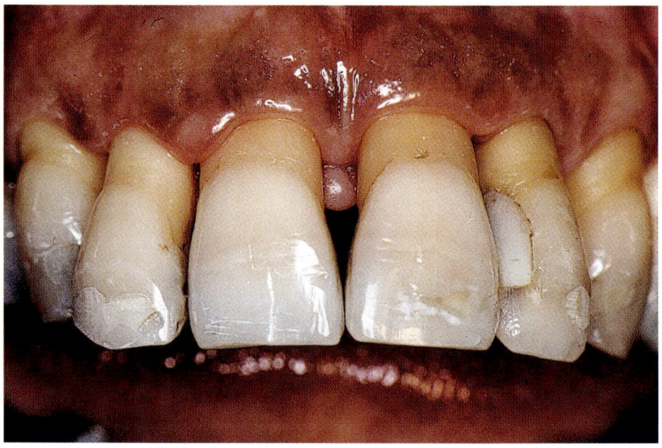

Fig 4-3f Two weeks postoperatively, periodontal stability has been achieved. When signs of disease are deemed to respond unsatisfactorily to treatment, additional treatment is always justified.

When deep pockets, bony lesions, or residual bony craters are present, corrective surgical management is indicated. The elimination of interproximal bony craters allows for better apical repositioning of soft tissues and greater pocket reduction than with nonosseous periodontal surgery. In the case of isolated, deep osseous lesions, regeneration or grafting techniques should be preferred.

A surgical approach is necessary for treatment of advanced periodontitis and stabilizes the results achieved through etiologic treatment (anti-infective and mechanical) (Figs 4-3a to 4-3f).

When the patient feels fully involved in treatment progress, surgery is perceived as a reward to diligent compliance to treatment recommendations:

- Successful achievement of the etiologic phase is validated through the decision to proceed to the surgical phase.
- When performed on healthy tissue, the surgical procedure is not painful and does not cause any secondary discomfort, and healing is quick.
- Esthetic consequences are predictable, and surgery of the anterior quadrant does not aggravate the damage caused by periodontal disease. In some cases surgery can even reduce it.

The practitioner has the satisfaction of having established the favorable conditions necessary to guide the patient through the treatment plan to the reevaluation phase.

Evaluation of surgical outcome (3 months postoperatively):
- Reduced pocket depth and presence of attachment gain (probing)
- Absence of bleeding on probing
- Elimination of pathogenic bacteria (microbiologic control test/probe/screening)
- Reduced plaque rate
- Radiographic evaluation

Effects of Antiseptic Medications

Mechanical treatment alone is often sufficient during initial therapy. To improve the outcome of nonsurgical treatment, and if antimicrobial control is insufficient, use of topical antimicrobial agents can be a good option. Chlorhexidine mouthwashes are the most commonly used antiseptic solutions (concentrations range from 0.10% to 0.12%).

Efficacy of chlorhexidine has been verified in multiple clinical settings, and chlorhexidine remains the most prescribed antiseptic. It is also indicated as a complement to antibiotic therapy and as a postoperative antiseptic.

However, the following should be noted: chlorhexidine 0.2% has no effect on the biofilm when exposure is brief. Bactericidal activity of antiseptics is achieved through highly concentrated application for prolonged periods of time, eg, 2% chlorhexidine for 10 minutes to eradicate *P gingivalis*. Diffusion of these compounds into deep pockets is poorly controlled and disappointing overall. The biofilm is fully renewed after 6 days.

Prolonged use of chlorhexidine mouthwashes can lead to tooth discoloration, which can be discouraging for the patient (Figs 4-4a and 4-4b). During postoperative care, or when plaque control is reduced over short periods of time, antiseptic solutions may be applied locally with a surgical brush or gel; this allows for controlled delivery of antiseptic compound over a longer period of time.

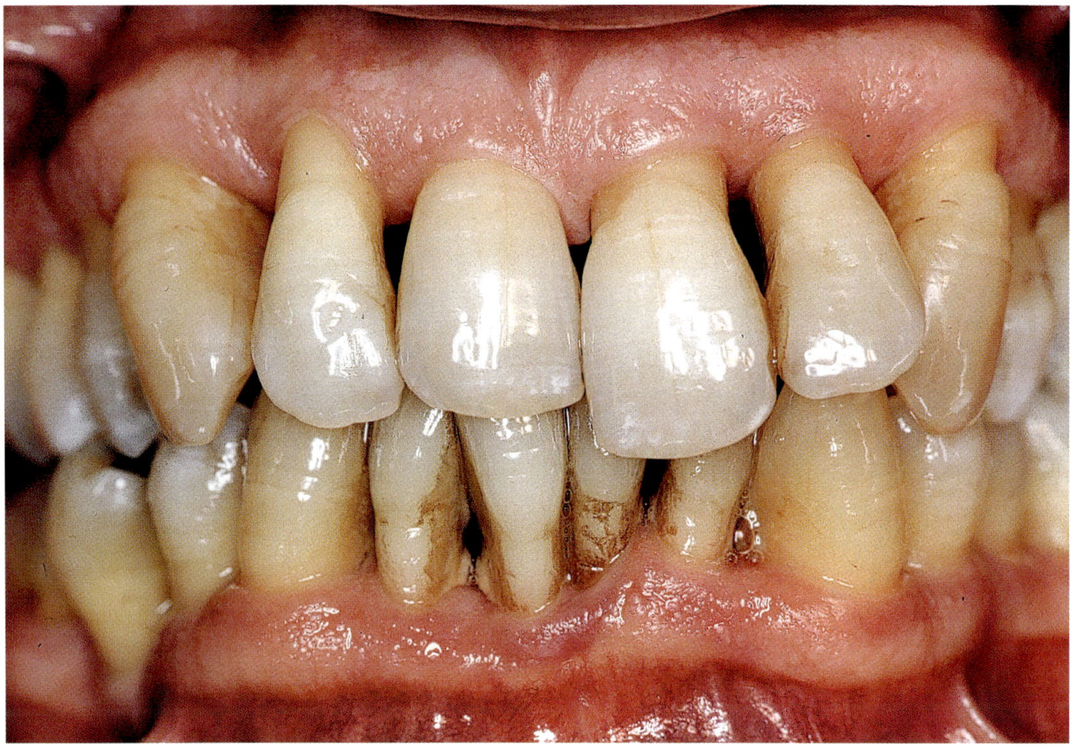

Fig 4-4a Severe aggressive periodontitis in a 46-year-old male patient.

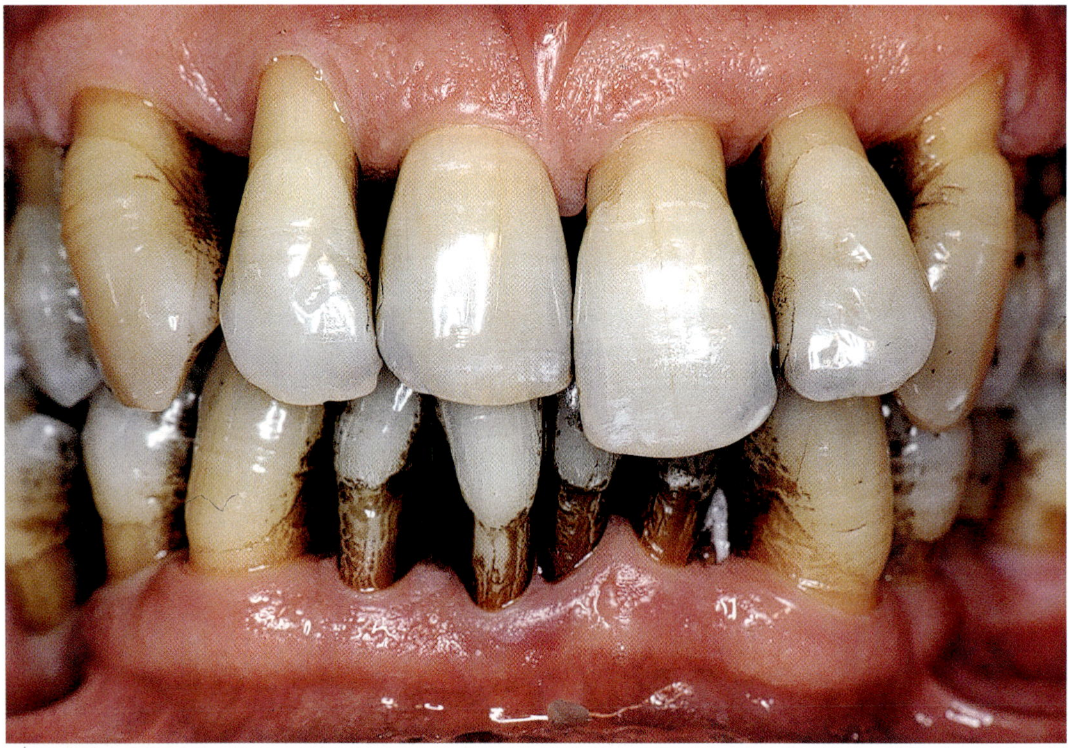

Fig 4-4b Marked tooth discoloration caused by chlorhexidine-based mouthwashes is often poorly accepted by patients. Fortunately this is easily eliminated.

Plaque-Induced Gingivitis

Plaque-induced gingivitis has been defined by the American Academy of Periodontology (2000) as a gingival inflammation occurring without clinical attachment loss. It is characterized by the presence of one of the following clinical signs: redness, swelling of gingival tissue, bleeding on probing, alteration of gingival contour and tissue appearance, presence of plaque and calculus, and absence of radiographic signs of bone loss. Presence of gingivitis does not systematically lead to periodontitis. However, it may be difficult to differentiate patients with gingivitis from those with periodontitis. Therefore, to reduce the prevalence of periodontitis, it is crucial to treat gingivitis systematically, particularly for patients in younger age categories, which are characterized by a higher prevalence of gingivitis.

The goal of treatment is restoration of gingival health through elimination of etiologic factors, including plaque, calculus, and other factors involved in plaque retention (Figs 4-5a and 4-5b). Clinical signs of gingival healing (eg, change in color, reduced swelling) appear quickly, while histologic signs (decrease in cellular and humoral inflammatory markers, tissue reorganization) are seen in later stages of the healing process (Brecx et al 1988).

This observation implies that treatment results should be assessed after a sufficient amount of time, in order to avoid rapid recurrence. This same concept probably applies to management of periodontitis.

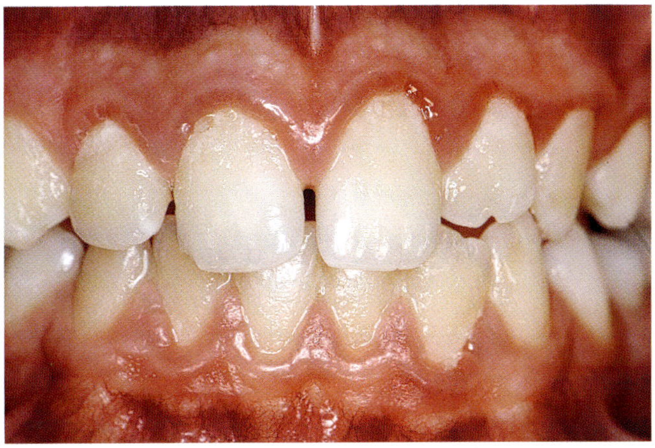

Fig 4-5a In this 12-year-old female patient, plaque scores are high. Gingivitis is directly related to the presence of plaque.

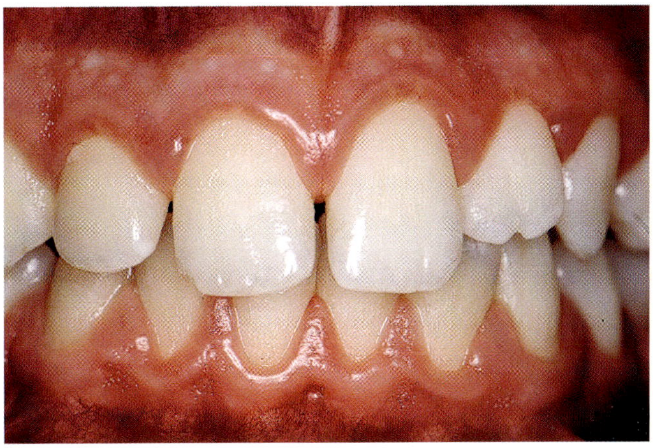

Fig 4-5b Oral hygiene instructions are immediately followed by one session of root scaling and planing. Subsequent monitoring of brushing efficiency leads to quick reversal of inflammation.

Treatment of Advanced Periodontitis

5

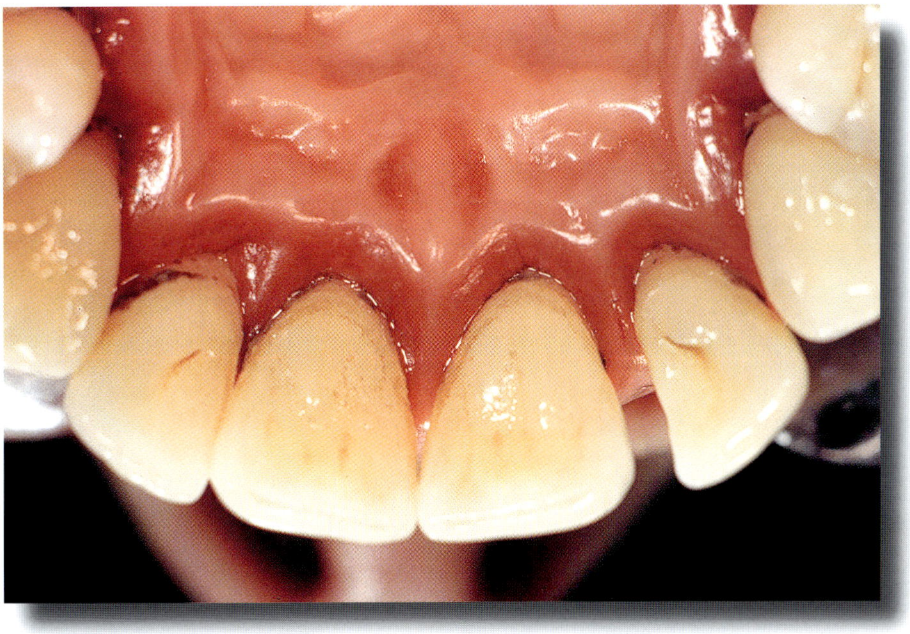

Chronic Periodontitis

Marginal chronic periodontitis

Similar to gingivitis, mild chronic periodontitis is induced by bacterial plaque; it is defined as gingival inflammation associated with clinical attachment loss less than one third of the root length. In the molar region, furcation invasion does not exceed Class I. Treatment is the same as that for gingivitis. After treatment, residual pockets and attachment loss are less than 4 mm, and as a general rule, surgical treatment is not necessary.

Marginal chronic periodontitis (pockets less than 4 mm) can usually be managed by scaling and root planing in a single treatment phase (Figs 5-1a and 5-1b).

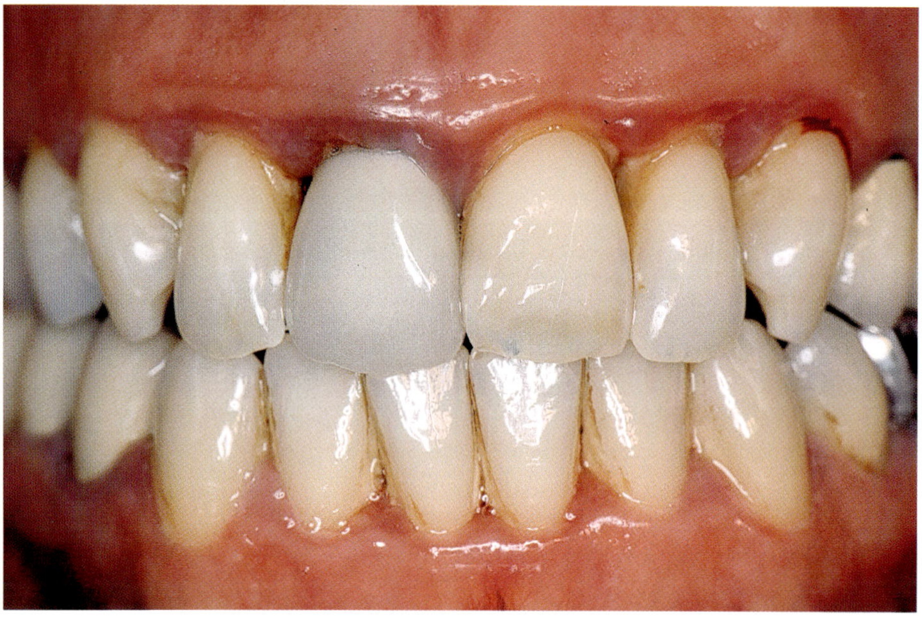

Fig 5-1a Mild chronic periodontitis in a 30-year-old, otherwise healthy patient. Generalized inflammation is associated with significant amounts of plaque and subgingival deposits. Infection involves a commensal-type flora.

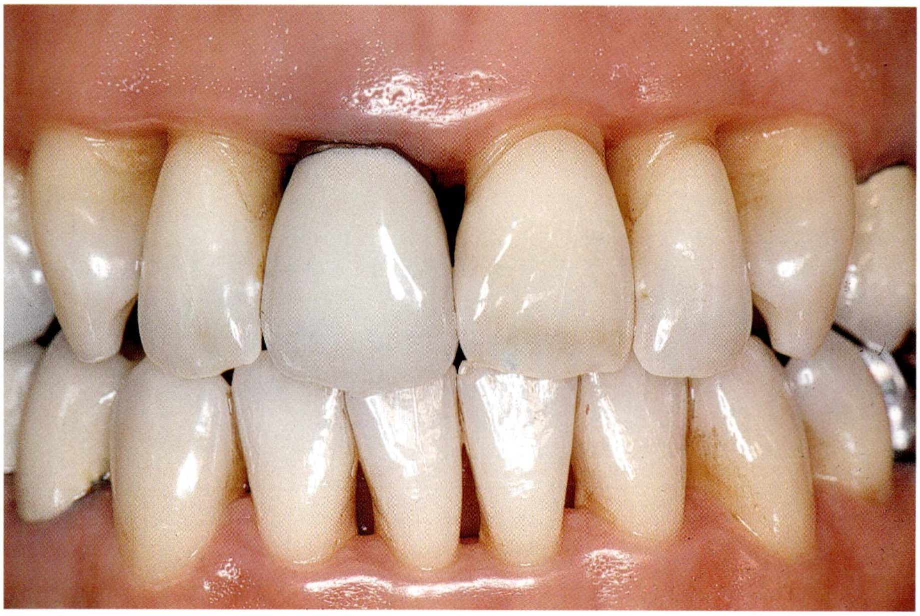

Fig 5-1b Periodontal therapy consists of oral hygiene instructions followed by two scaling and then two root planing sessions. Swift response to treatment occurs, with complete reversal of inflammation. There is a slight gingival recession, along with papillae tissue loss. As a general rule, surgery is not necessary; it may, however, be indicated when bony defects are present or to improve gingival conditions before prosthetic care.

Moderate to locally advanced chronic periodontitis

Moderate chronic periodontitis (once known as *adult periodontitis*) is the most common form of periodontitis. It occurs in all age groups. It is characterized by a slow progression with intermittent periods of rapid progression (American Academy of Periodontology 2000).

Clinical signs and symptoms

- Swelling, redness, and bleeding on probing are present, with or without suppuration.
- Chronic periodontitis is qualified as moderate when loss of periodontal attachment is greater than or equal to one third of the root length. Probing depth may reach 6 mm and clinical attachment loss 4 mm. Increased mobility is often observed. In the furcae, attachment loss does not exceed Class I.
- Radiographic evaluation displays evidence of bone loss.
- Moderate chronic periodontitis may be localized to one tooth, extend to several teeth, or be generalized to all quadrants. Simultaneously in a given patient, there may be healthy areas and other areas featuring chronic periodontitis with slight, moderate, or severe levels of destruction.

Treatment goals

Treatment goals involve controlling or eliminating microbial factors altogether, as well as modifying risk factors to arrest disease progression durably. Periodontal health and functional and esthetic comfort must subsequently be maintained and recurrence prevented. Commensal infection is preponderant. Therefore, local treatment is the priority since it reduces bacterial load and may promote a bacterial equilibrium that is compatible with periodontal health. The reduction of inflammatory signs is a hallmark for these microbiologic changes. Locally, an attempt at regenerating the attachment system may be made.

Several different factors may affect treatment planning and the general outcome: some are patient-related and include general health status, age, motivation, cooperation, and plaque-control proficiency. Other factors include the clinician's ability to eliminate subgingival deposits, the need for dental and prosthetic work, and the presence of sites with severe periodontal destruction.

Conventional treatment

Initial treatment (etiologic)

- Systemic risk factors (diabetes, systemic disease), behavior-related risk factors (smoking), environment-related risk factors (stress), or bacterial risk factors (presence of virulent pathogenic species) are likely to compromise success of conventional treatment. These factors should be properly controlled or eliminated when possible.
- Oral hygiene instructions, improvement, and assessment of plaque control.
- Supra- and subgingival scaling and root planing.
- Eventually, administration of antimicrobial agents (antibiotics and antiseptics).
- Elimination or correction of local, iatrogenic, or functional risk factors.
- Assessment of initial treatment phase outcome. This involves screening through all disease markers. An appropriate time interval should be respected, to allow for tissue repair and a reduction of inflammation to occur. Three different possibilities should be anticipated:
  - Outcome is unsatisfactory because of poor plaque control. Chances for treatment success are slim to none.

- Outcome is satisfactory, and stable periodontal health has been achieved. The patient is placed in supportive/maintenance therapy.
- Outcome is satisfactory as far as inflammation is concerned, but the conditions necessary to achieve stable periodontal health have not been established. Adjunct treatment should be considered (surgery or other).

Periodontal surgery

- Periodontal augmentation surgery
- Corrective surgery
  - Flap surgery with or without ostectomy
  - Prosthetic surgical preparation prior to prosthetic rehabilitation
- Reparative surgery
  - Bone grafts
  - Guided tissue regeneration
  - Combined techniques

Other treatments

- Resume some aspects of initial therapy
- Correct other risk factors (cessation of smoking, systemic disease management)
- Establish a periodontal maintenance schedule

Conditions required for therapeutic success

The predictable effects of a successful conventional treatment for mild or moderate chronic periodontitis are:

- A decrease in plaque to a level compatible with gingival health
- A significant reduction of all clinical signs of inflammation
- Pocket depth reduction
- Stability or, at best, clinical attachment gain

In areas where tissue response is poor, the following items may be observed:

- Persistence of residual inflamed gingival tissue
- Persistence or increase in pocket depth for deep pockets
- Unstable clinical attachment levels
- Persistent plaque rates to a degree incompatible with gingival health

Frequently, localized areas display persistent signs of instability, though the general periodontal context displays overall improvement of disease markers. In these cases, specific adjunct therapy should be considered.

Case report of moderate chronic periodontitis with locally advanced sites

Forty-one-year-old, otherwise healthy, nonsmoking female patient, brushes twice a day and uses toothpicks. Family history reveals that the patient's mother was edentulous at age 45 (Figs 5-2a to 5-2bb).

Chief complaints

Tooth mobility, pain on chewing in maxillary incisors and right first molar; long history of bleeding gingiva.

Clinical signs

Halitosis, inflammation (most prominent in lingual/palatal aspects of all quadrants), bacterial plaque, calculus, attachment loss (generally 4 to 6 mm, locally 8 to 10 mm), pockets, dental mobility (Class II to IV), secondary diastemata, bone loss from one third to two thirds of the root length, furcation invasion and presence of angular lesions, primary anterior overbite, absence of canine guidance, improperly fitting restorations, molar occlusal trauma, lingual hyperfunction.

Severity

Moderate to severe; attachment losses frequently exceed 6 mm.

Complexity factors

These are essentially local factors, such as plaque, restorations, functional occlusal disorder, and overload. Destruction is linked to the presence of these local factors.

Diagnosis

Moderate to severe chronic periodontitis featuring a predominant endogenous-type infection, caused by growth of a selected number of commensal anaerobic populations, and aggravated by numerous local factors.

Treatment goals and methods

The chief objective is to control infection and to eliminate inflammation; this is achieved through proper plaque control, placement of provisional restorations, and scaling and root planing. Progressive reduction or disappearance of inflammation indicates a favorable evolution in treatment; inflammatory signs (swelling, redness, bleeding) are reversible, while those related to destruction (horizontal bone loss) are not. Some improvement (attachment gains, reduction of probing depths, dental mobility, migration) is nevertheless likely to occur.

Periodontal treatment generally leads to reduction or correction of dental displacement, occasionally without further indication for orthodontic therapy. Orthodontic treatment, if initiated too early, may render assessment of the response potential difficult.

Restorative periodontal strategies aim at eliminating complexity factors (ill-fitting restorations) and risk factors (pockets).

It seems unlikely in this clinical case that a course of antibiotic therapy will be necessary.

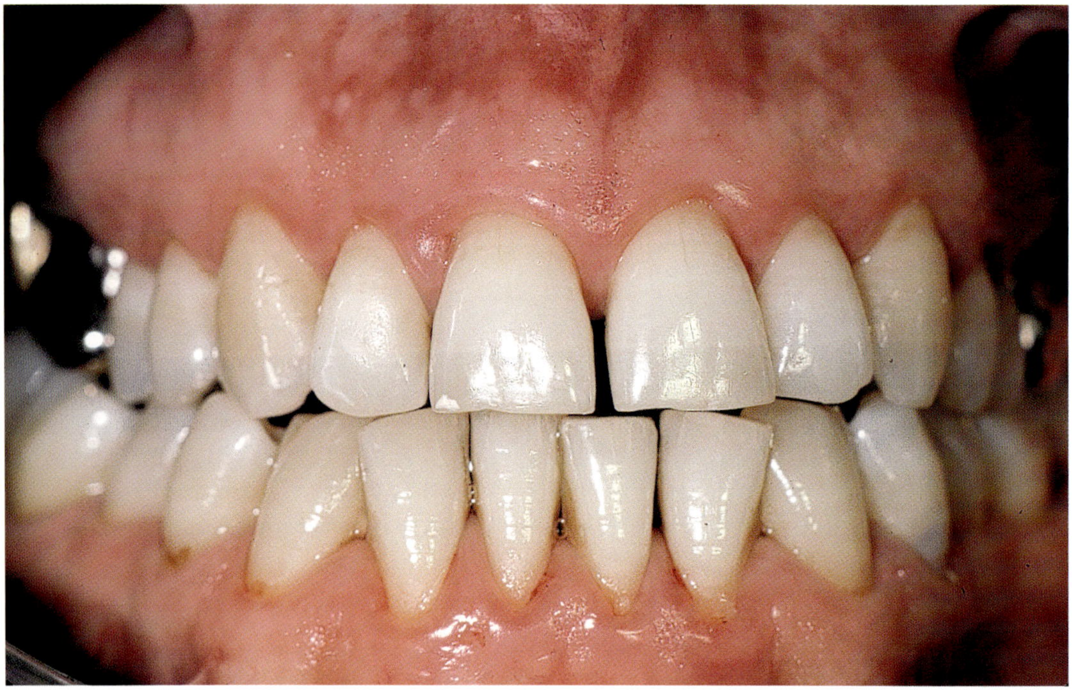

Fig 5-2a Moderate to severe periodontitis in a 41-year-old female patient. Inflammation is mild on the facial aspect of the gingiva. Tooth migrations and diastemata have recently occurred. The maxillary right central incisor presents Class III mobility. There is an anterior open bite.

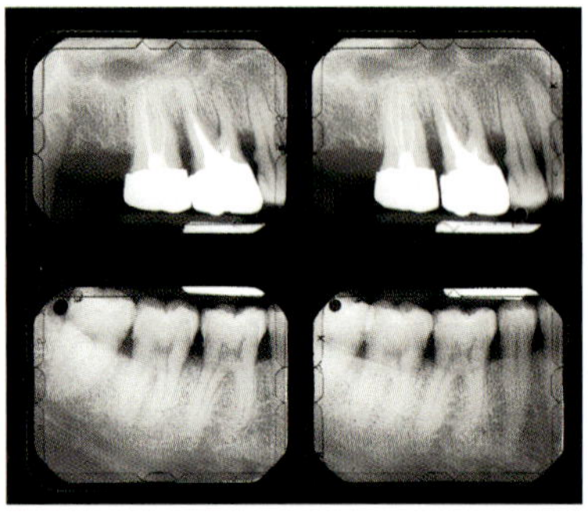

Fig 5-2b Bone loss is more significant around prosthetically restored maxillary molars, especially the right first molar.

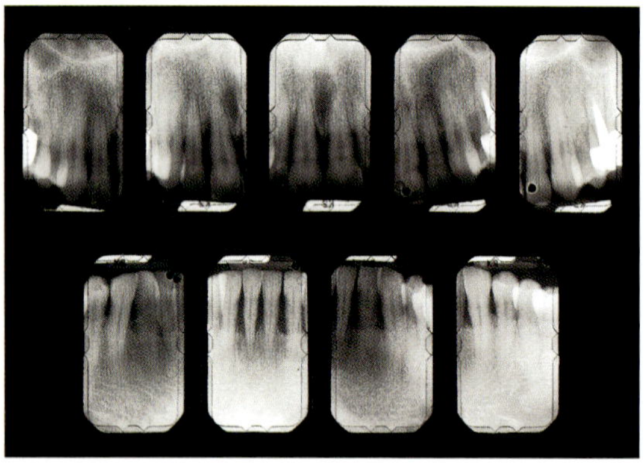

Fig 5-2c Bone destruction is irregularly distributed. In some places, it reaches 50%.

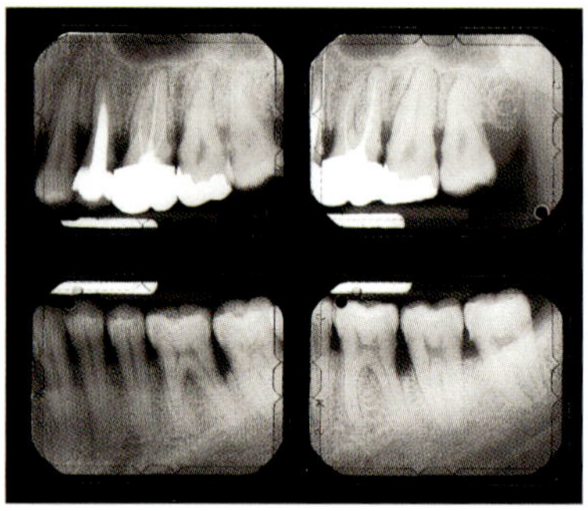

Fig 5-2d Here again, bone destruction is more advanced in restored teeth (maxillary left second premolar, first molar, and second molar). Mandibular teeth present less bone destruction. Severity factors are local and functional in nature.

Risk factors

Bacterial plaque, a possible predisposition to periodontal disease, and presence of persistent periodontal pockets are a few of the risk factors.

Recurrent subgingival bacterial colonization increases the likelihood of disease progression. This risk is directly proportional to the patient's ability to effectively control the accumulation of plaque, as well as to the persistence of high-risk sites, including deep pockets, furcation invasions, and mobile teeth.

Prognosis

Good.

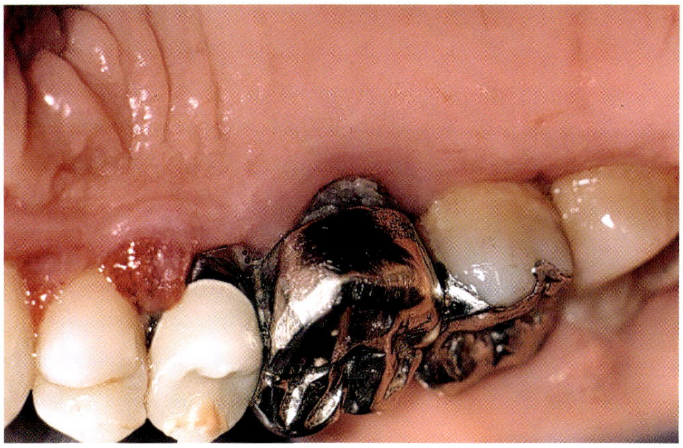

Fig 5-2e Clinical signs of inflammation are marked on the lingual/palatal aspects of restored teeth. Plaque control is unsatisfactory.

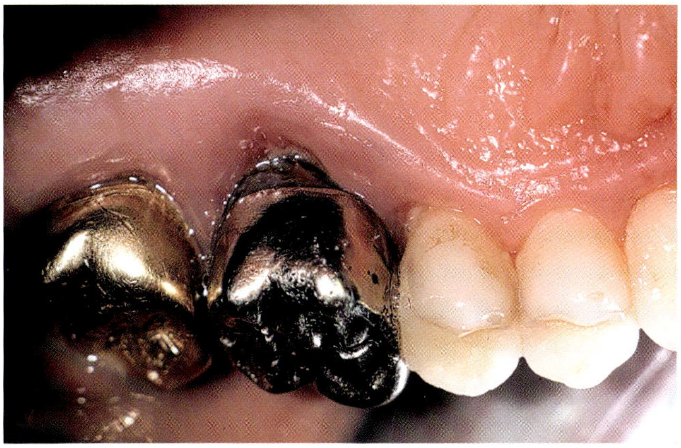

Fig 5-2f Attachment loss around the first molar exceeds 10 mm and involves the furcation. The tooth presents Class III mobility. The tooth is very tender to percussion.

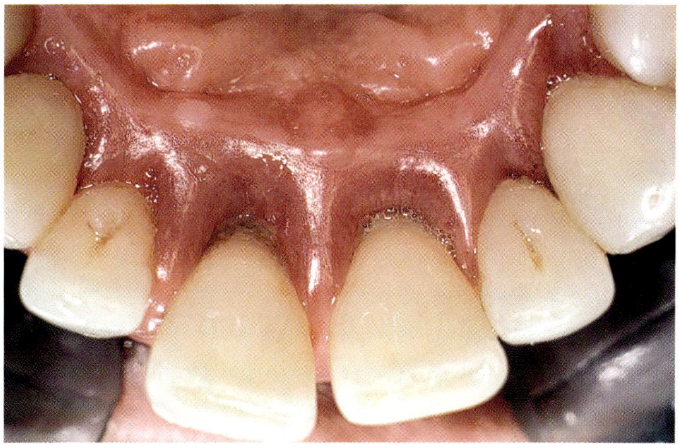

Fig 5-2g Significant amounts of plaque deposit are visible on the palatal aspect of the maxillary right central incisor. This evokes the characteristic aspect of plaque biofilm. Opposite the root surface, gingival recession has occurred concomitantly to intense inflammation. The maxillary right central incisor exhibits Class III or higher mobility. Attachment loss exceeds 10 mm on the distal aspect. Interincisal diastema is of recent onset (6 months).

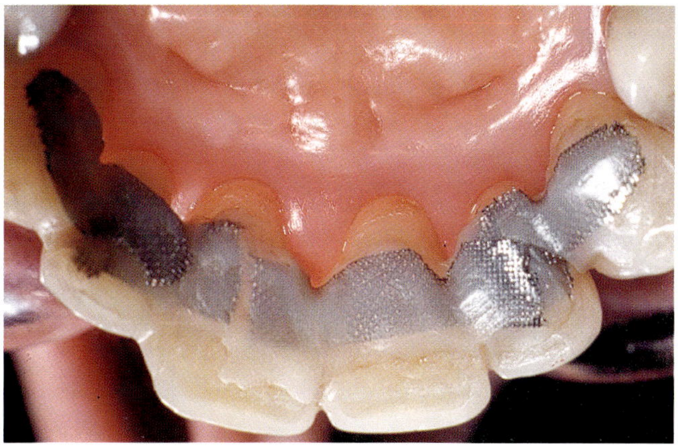

Fig 5-2h After two scaling sessions, two planing sessions, periodontal surgery, and orthodontic treatment, inflammation has disappeared and attachment gain has occurred around the incisors. Transitional splinting is performed on all six anterior teeth.

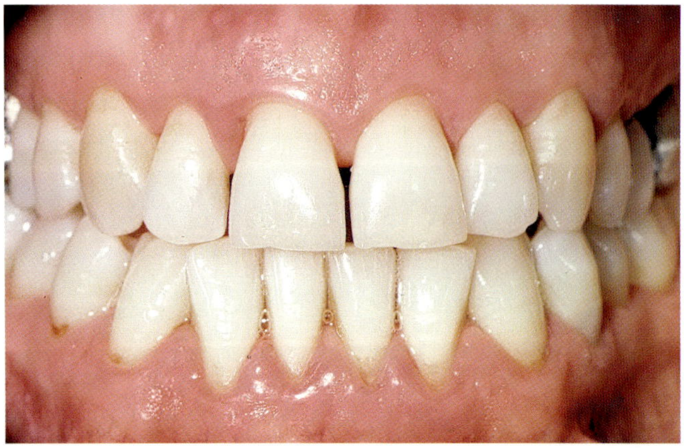

Fig 5-2i Plaque control and scaling and root planing sessions reduce inflammatory signs and lead to a significant, spontaneous reversal of the central diastema.

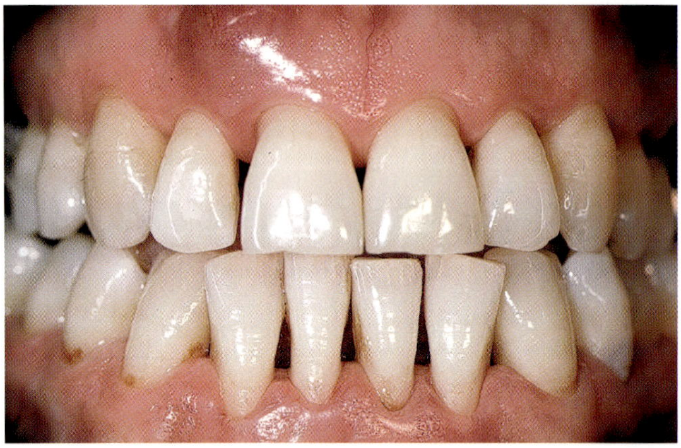

Fig 5-2j An infectious incident occurs after root planing. The bacterial balance is modified. The elimination of residual beneficial species promotes tissue invasion by residual pathogens. Note the quick closure of the diastema subsequent to an inflammatory episode: a change in inflammatory status may artificially reduce secondary migrations.

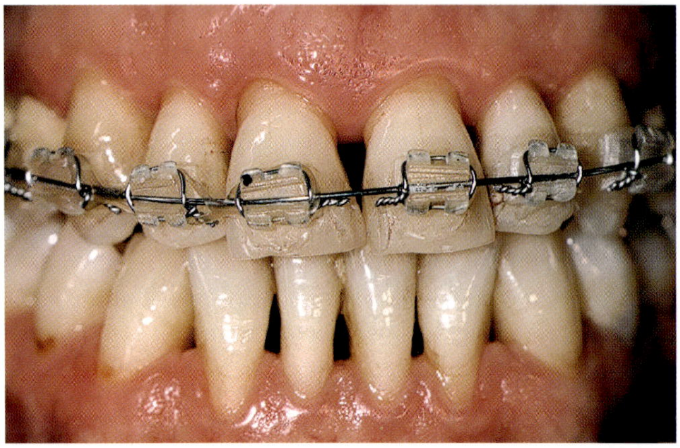

Fig 5-2k Antibiotic treatment is necessary (amoxicillin 500 mg tid for 8 days and metronidazole 500 mg tid for 8 days). Periodontal flap surgery is performed. Orthodontic treatment is performed to reverse residual diastemata and restore canine guidance.

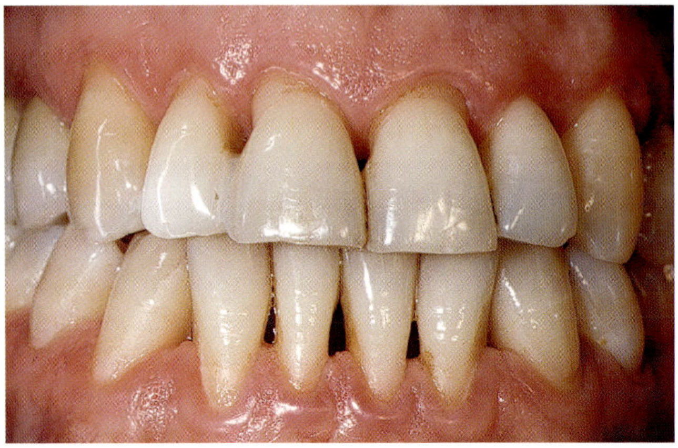

Fig 5-2l Active treatment is finished. Anterior open bite is reduced and canine guidance restored. Occlusal rehabilitation of posterior regions can begin.

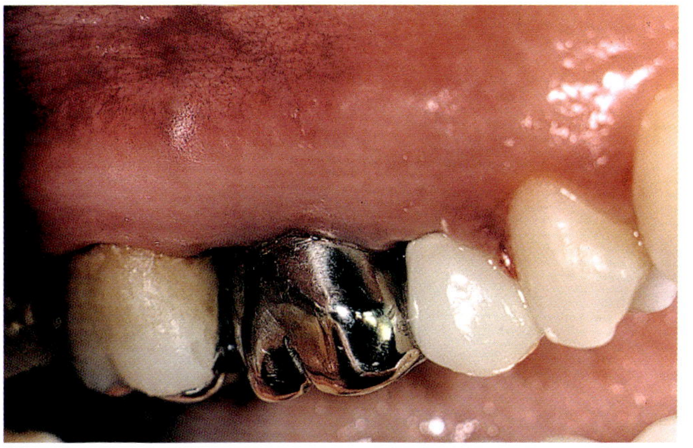

Fig 5-2m Here again, inflammation is significant and features spontaneous bleeding. Proximal attachment losses exhibit probing depths ranging from 4 to 6 mm and extend to molar furcation regions (Class I). An open bite exists between the first molar and the antagonist tooth.

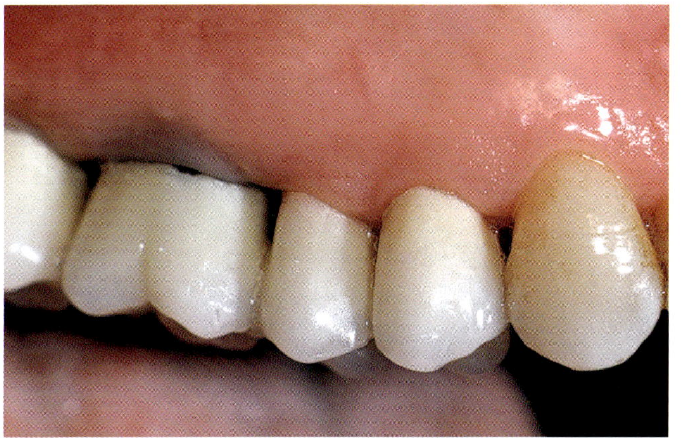

Fig 5-2n Inflammation is reduced through plaque control and scaling and root planing. Provisional crowns are placed on all molars and premolars. Residual probing depths range from 4 to 6 mm. Interdental hygiene needs to be perfected.

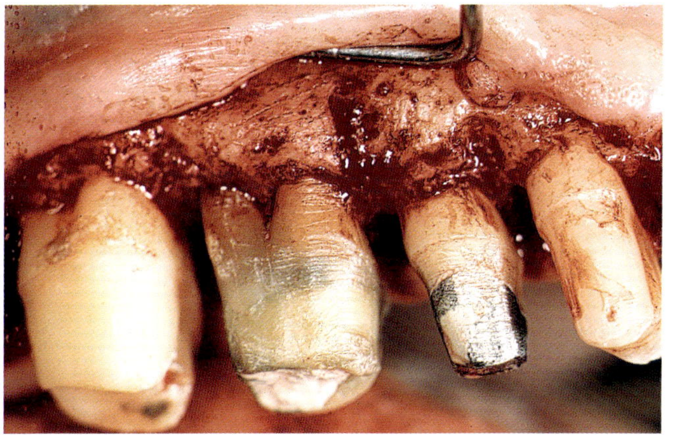

Fig 5-2o Periodontal surgery is carried out to improve root planing, reduce residual pockets, correct bone contour by osteoplasty, correct interproximal bony craters, improve plaque control in furcation regions, extract the third molar, and prepare dental prosthetic conditions for further rehabilitation.

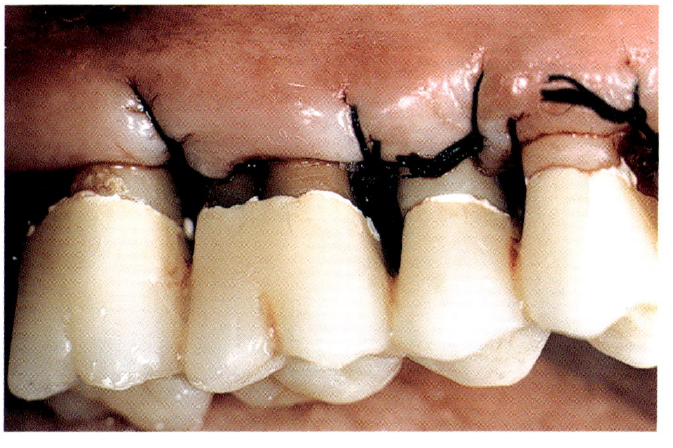

Fig 5-2p Apical flap repositioning achieves a 3-mm crown lengthening. Temporary surgical dressing is left in place for 5 to 7 days to allow for hygiene measures to be performed (this involved a surgical brush dipped in a chlorhexidine solution). Conditions propitious to first-line healing must be achieved.

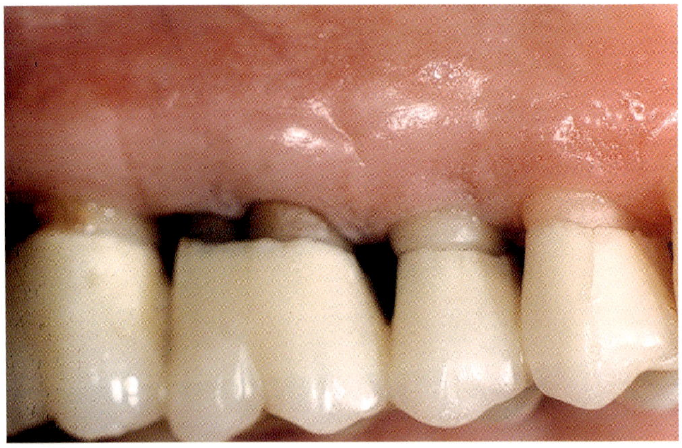

Fig 5-2q Once sutures are removed, root planing is performed 3 and 5 weeks postoperatively. Proximal cleaning with interdental brushes is possible in this new clinical situation. Note the quality of healing.

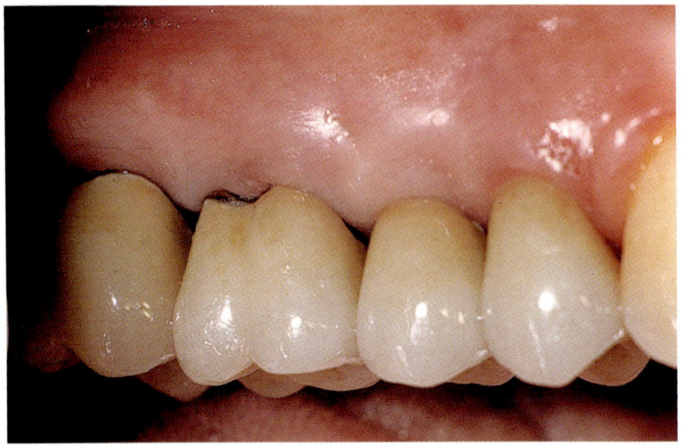

Fig 5-2r Prosthetic restorations are in place. Note the quality of relationship between the gingival tissue and the restorations. The furcation region of the prosthetic profile (the marked depression of the restoration) allows for easy access of plaque control procedures in this area.

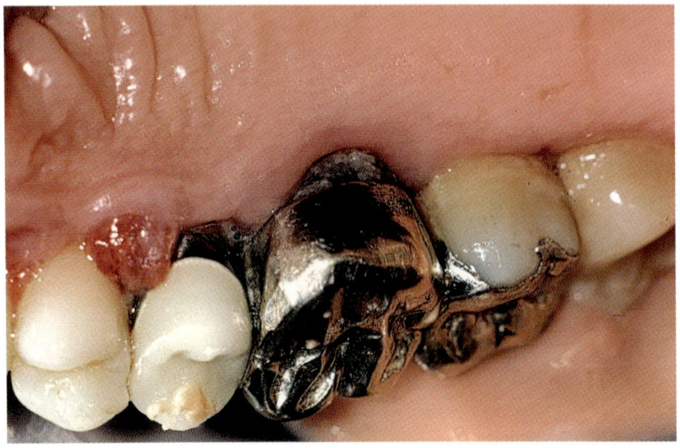

Fig 5-2s In the premolar region, budding of inflammatory tissue marks the presence of local plaque-retaining factors (ill-fitting crown and narrow interdental space).

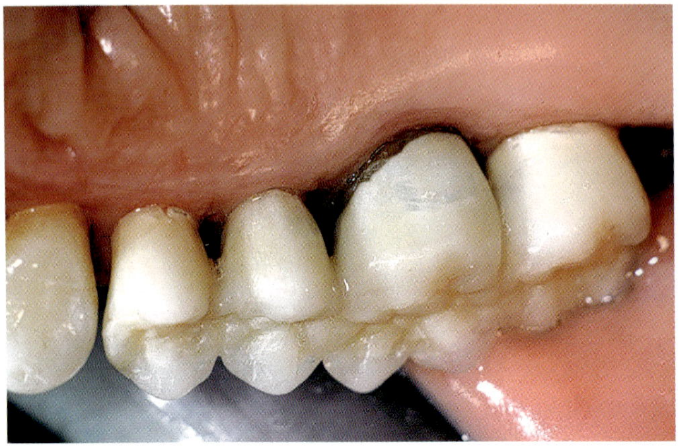

Fig 5-2t At reevaluation, the achievement of initial objectives is evaluated: plaque control, reduction of inflammation and bleeding, modification of plaque-retaining factors, and improvement of attachment levels. The need for additional treatment is also assessed.

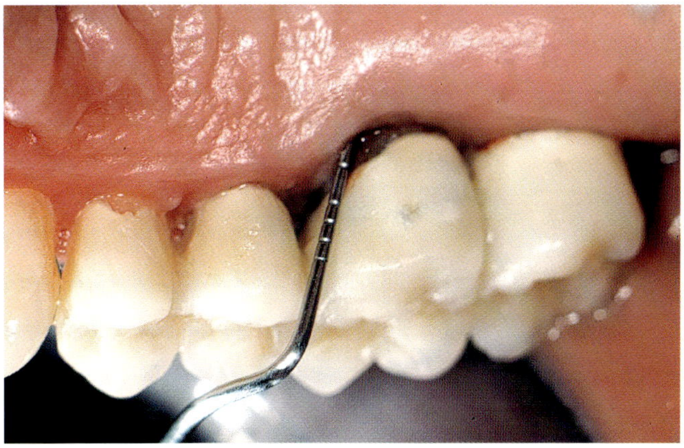

Fig 5-2u As a general rule, surgery is not required in areas where probing depths are less than 4 mm. However, when global periodontal management involves prosthetic rehabilitation, surgery should be considered.

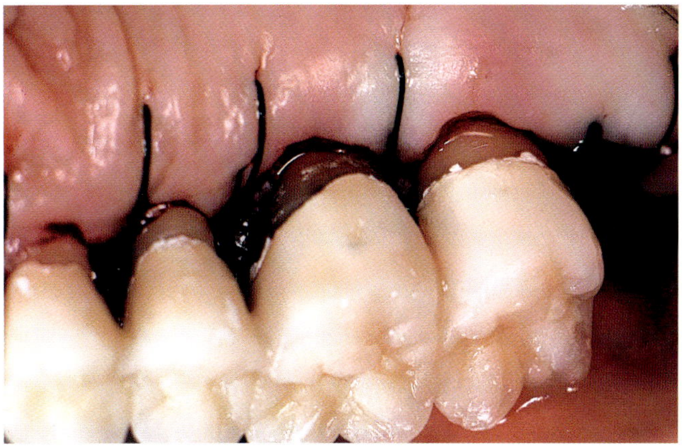

Fig 5-2v Apical flap repositioning is impossible on the palatal aspect. Flap design is defined by the primary incision. The suture holds the flap tightly adapted around teeth. The resulting crown lengthening is approximately 3 mm.

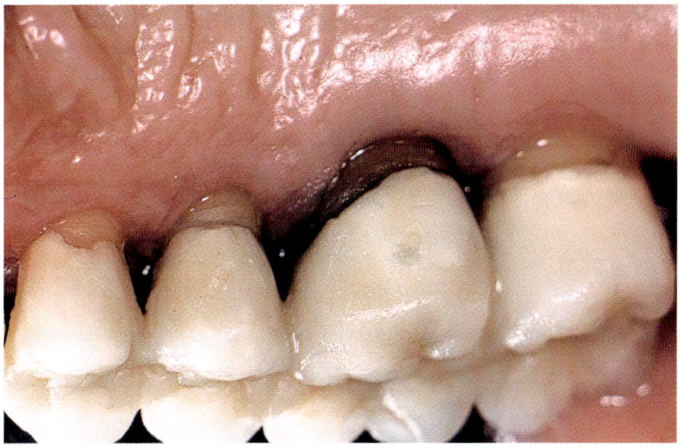

Fig 5-2w After healing, there is no need to precipitate prosthetic recontouring. It is often necessary to wait more than 8 weeks to obtain optimal gingival repair (epithelial-connective tissue attachment, new gingival sulcus, absence of postsurgical proximal craters).

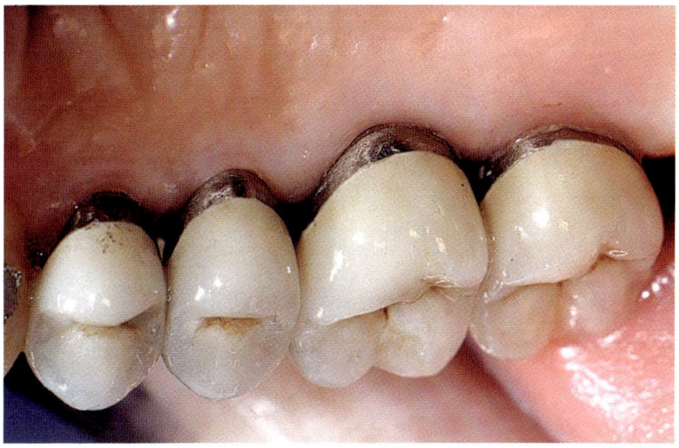

Fig 5-2x Final prosthetic restorations in place. Note favorable gingival healing (compare with Fig 5-2s).

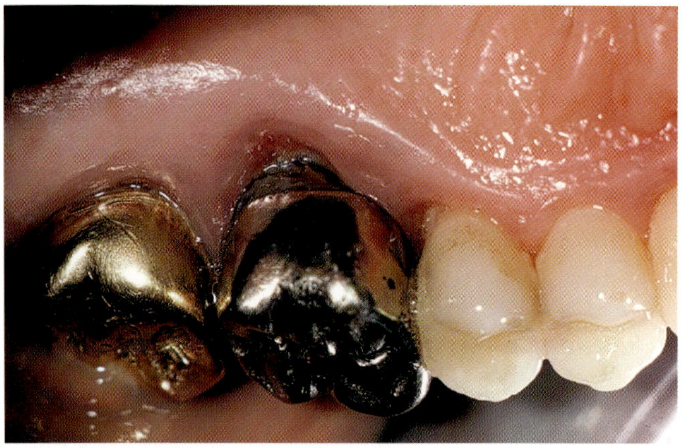

Fig 5-2y In the opposite maxillary quadrant, preoperative clinical signs around the first molar are severe: the tooth exhibits Class III mobility and is very tender to pressure.

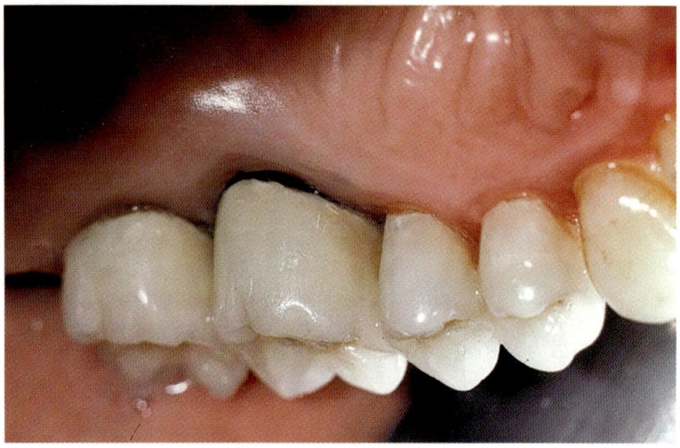

Fig 5-2z Provisional restorations have facilitated plaque removal and contributed to restoration of functional balance. They are an integral part of initial treatment. Endodontic treatments are initiated at this point.

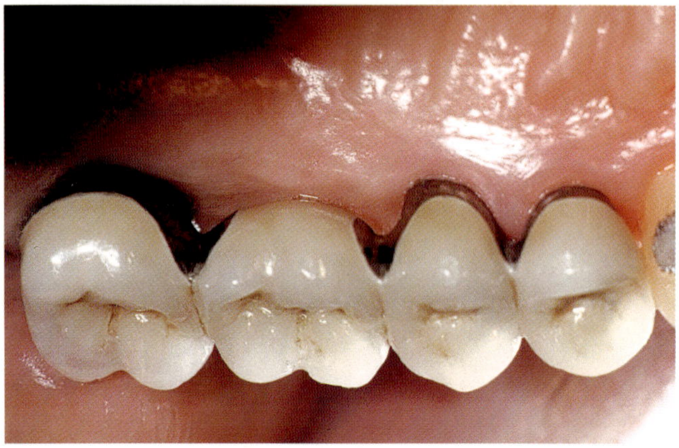

Fig 5-2aa The first molar was extracted because of a longitudinal fracture. Note the periodontal profile of the prosthetic restorations.

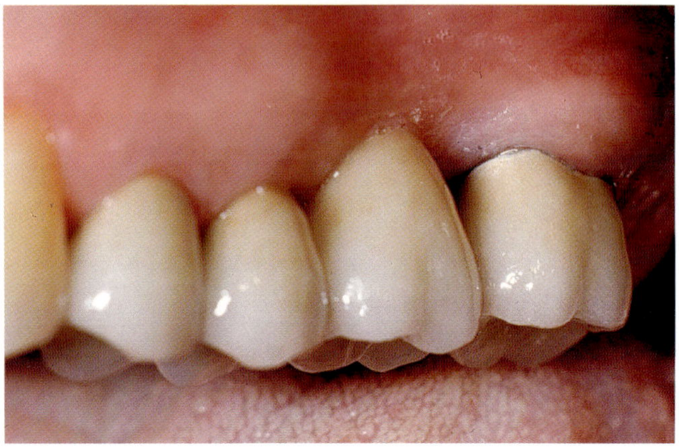

Fig 5-2bb Conditions for successful treatment—favorable hygiene conditions, elimination of infection (that is, all signs of inflammation have disappeared), correction of local severity factors, pocket reduction, and attachment stability—have been achieved.

Generalized advanced chronic periodontitis

Generalized advanced chronic periodontitis features clinical signs and treatment needs that are more significant than those encountered in moderate periodontitis. Treatment goals, conventional treatment, and conditions for success are similar (American Academy of Periodontology 2000). Clinical signs that are specific to advanced periodontitis include:

- Loss of periodontal support exceeding one third of the root length
- Furcation involvement showing Class II or III tissue destruction
- Probing depths exceeding 6 mm and attachment losses greater than 4 mm

Conventional treatment

Initial treatment

- Bacterial culture can be justified in specific sites where severe infection is present; this aims at identifying pathogenic species and at testing their sensitivity to the antibiotic regimen that is most likely to be administered.
- At this point in treatment, teeth with a poor prognosis should be extracted.
- Periodontal surgery; root amputation surgery may also be indicated.

Adjunctive treatment

When the patient is compliant with oral hygiene procedures, the outcome of root planing may be improved. Exposed root surfaces may be covered through local surgical measures.

Conditions for treatment success

- Adequate treatment planning
- Radiographic assessment of bone regeneration
- Restoration of functional and occlusal stability

Severity factors

In advanced chronic periodontitis, severity factors include bacterial plaque, smoking, and a host of local factors, such as plaque retention, presence of calculus, ill-fitting restorations, and functional factors. As a general rule, periodontal destruction is unevenly distributed throughout the dentition. This can be interpreted as a sign of host resistance that locally fails to overcome infection if, in addition, local risk factors are present. Correcting or reversing these local factors is a key point in periodontal treatment.

Implants and advanced periodontitis

Loss of teeth, or the decision to extract those that are severely compromised, will lead clinicians to define the different criteria for the use of implants in the management of periodontal disease (Fig 5-3).

Fig 5-3 A 54-year-old, otherwise healthy, nonsmoking male patient experiences significant pain and discomfort during masticatory function. The patient has given little care to his dentition in the past and has undergone no periodontal monitoring.

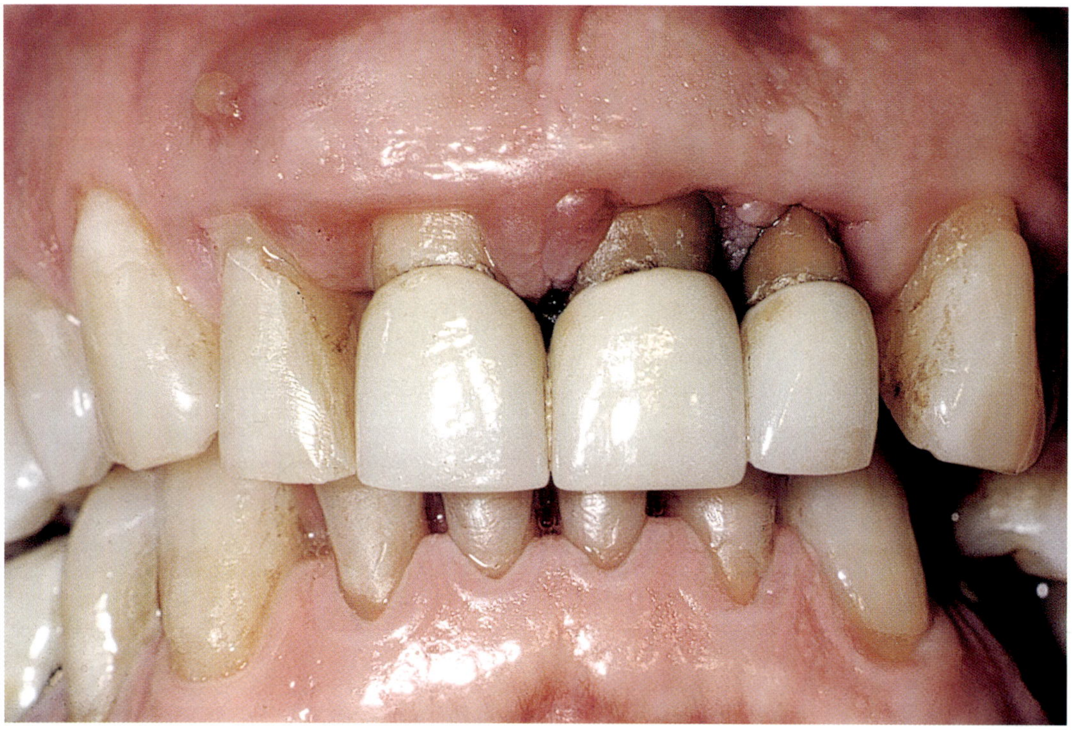

Fig 5-3a Severe inflammation and suppuration at maxillary incisors and canine teeth, along with marked functional occlusal disturbance (anterior overbite, maxillary incisor mobility) are evident. Periodontal tissue in the anterior mandibular region is within normal limits.

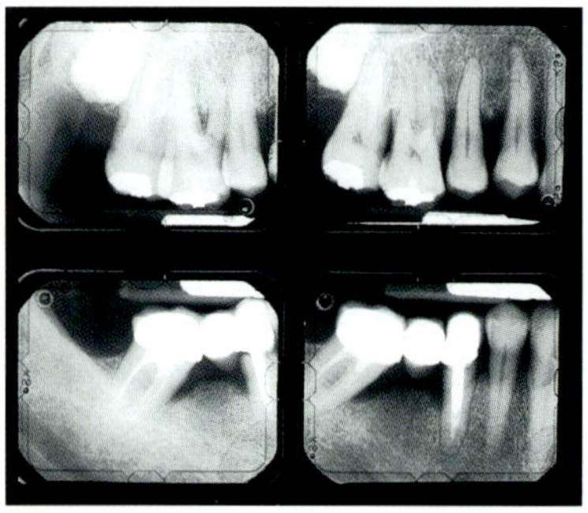

Fig 5-3b Bone destruction is moderate (greater than 5 mm) in the maxilla. In the mandible it is irregular, featuring angular lesions on the mesial aspect of the right second molar and the distal aspect of the right second premolar.

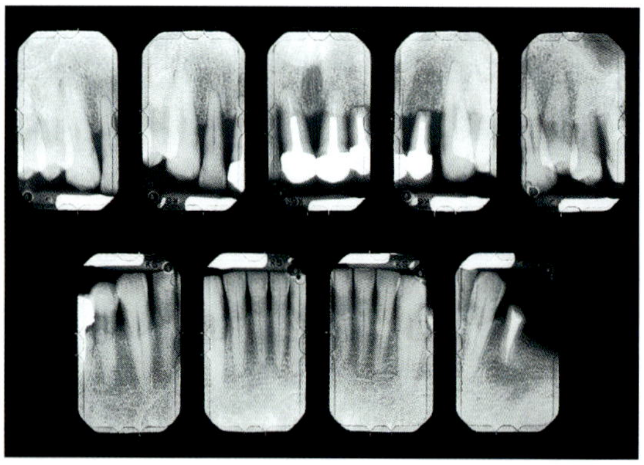

Fig 5-3c There is significant contrast between the degree of bone destruction in the anterior maxillary region, which displays terminal bone destruction and high probing depths, and mild destruction in the mandible.

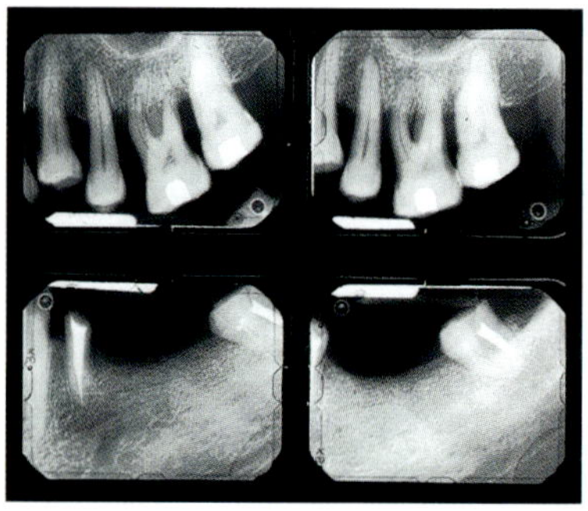

Fig 5-3d Tooth migration, mobility, and diastemata can be observed, as well as furcation bone loss around the maxillary left first molar; there is a significant edentulous region in the mandible.

The diagnosis is advanced chronic periodontitis with unevenly distributed degrees of severity. Where high degrees of severity are present (as in the maxilla) local factors are involved and are infectious, prosthetic, and functional in nature. Localized resistance, such as that found in the mandibular incisor region, indicates the patient's low susceptibility. Infection is commensal. Local severity factors are present. Prognosis is good on the condition that these local factors are eliminated.

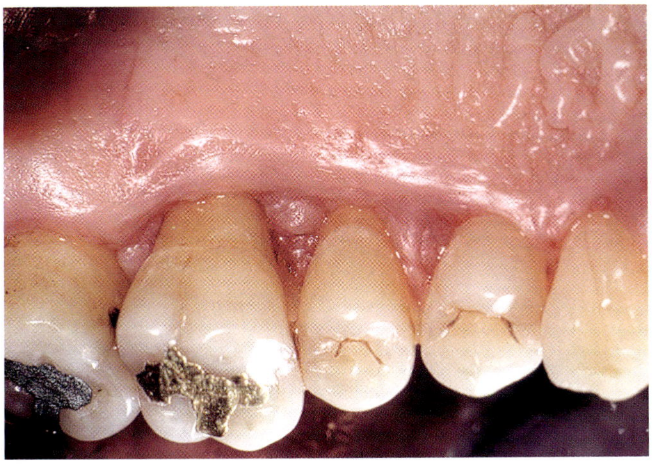

Fig 5-3e Clinical signs in the maxillary right posterior include inflammation, pockets, gingival craters, and attachment loss.

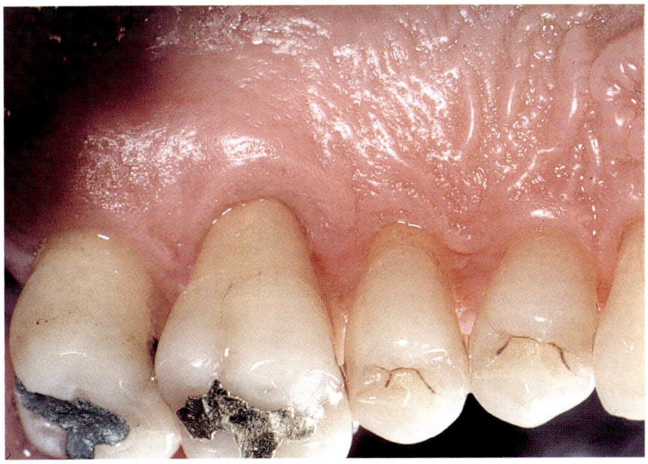

Fig 5-3f After treatment involving plaque control, scaling and root planing, and periodontal surgery for pocket depth reduction, periodontal tissues have recovered their normal aspect.

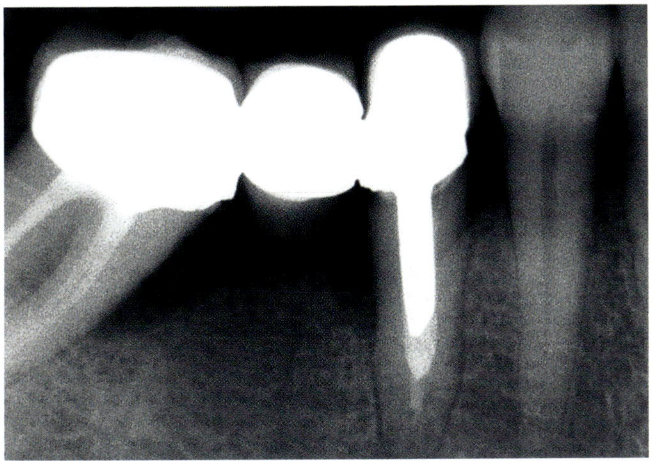

Fig 5-3g Attachment loss and deep pockets on the mesial aspect of the mandibular right second molar and distal aspect of the second premolar (angular lesions).

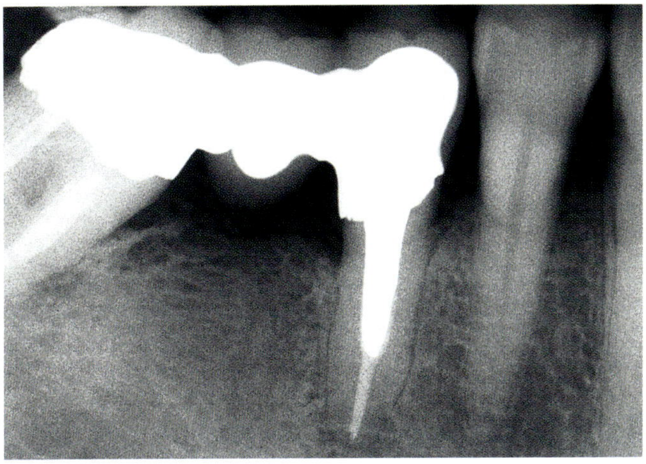

Fig 5-3h Eight years after grafting with tricalcic phosphate, these sites have achieved stability. Significant clinical attachment gains have been achieved as well as pocket depth reduction.

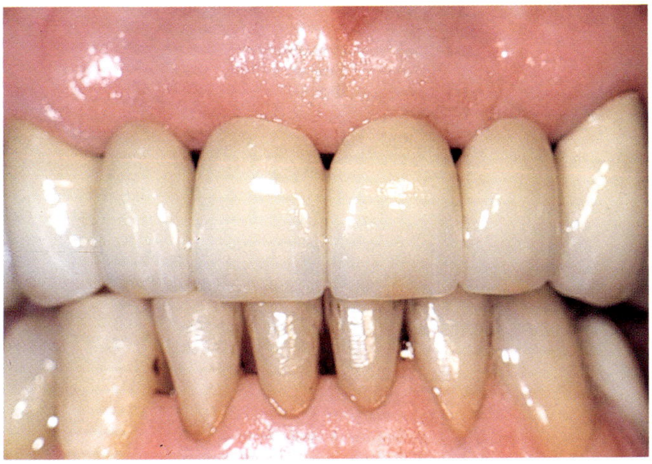

Fig 5-3i Pocket depth reduction is achieved after extraction of the maxillary incisors. A fixed partial denture allows for recovery of functional occlusal balance. Note the favorable response of the periodontal tissue.

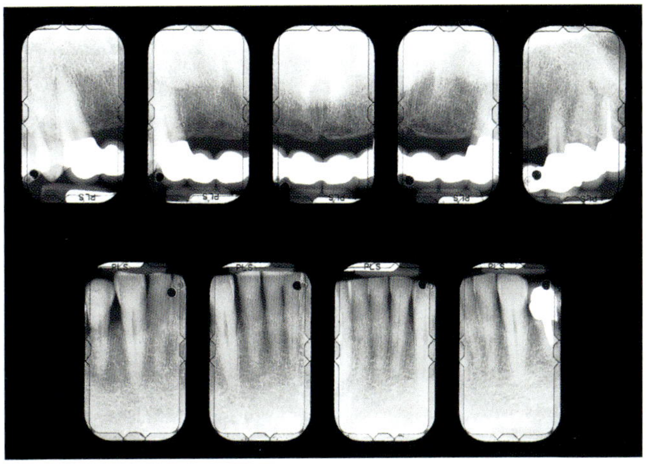

Fig 5-3j Periodontal bone tissues are stable.

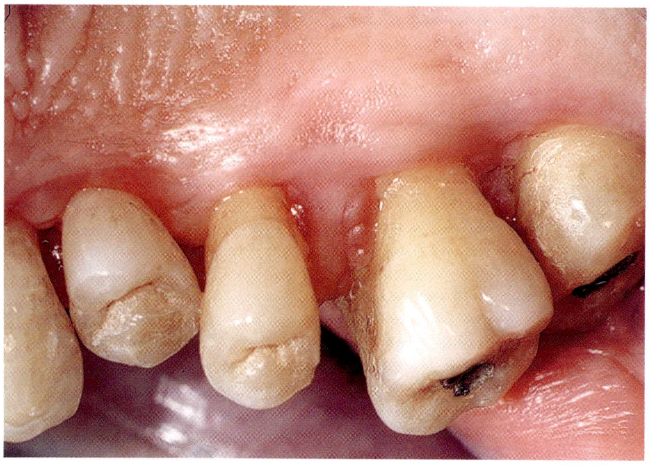

Fig 5-3k Clinical signs in the maxillary left posterior region include inflammation, periodontal pockets, attachment loss, and loss of interproximal contacts.

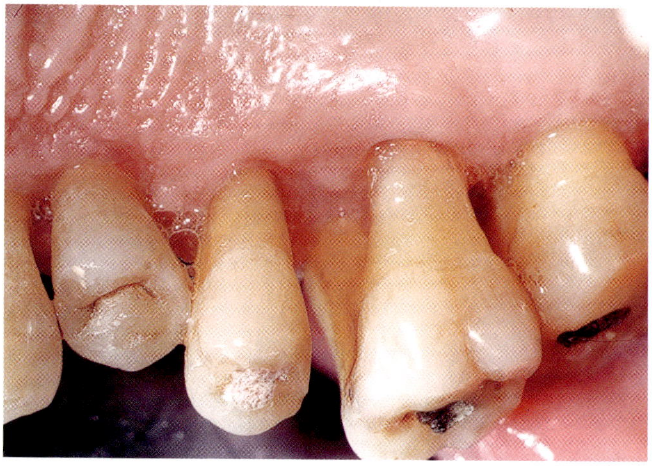

Fig 5-3l Treatment of infection (plaque control, prophylaxis, scaling and root planing) and periodontal surgery are performed before extraction of the first molar. This is done to eliminate a high-risk site.

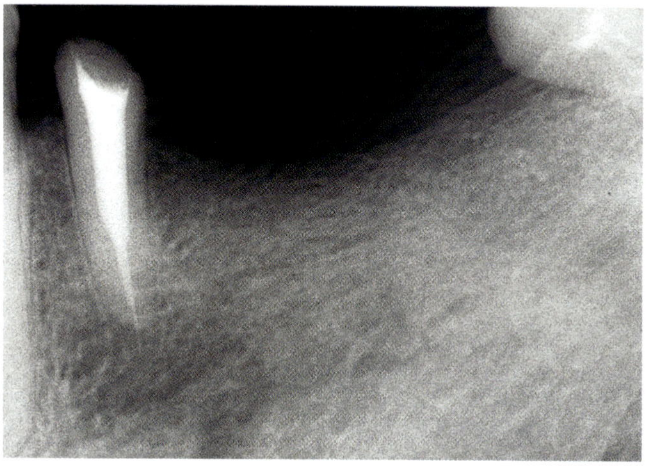

Fig 5-3m Treatment of a partially edentulous region can be oriented toward an implant-based solution. Placement of implants is performed once infectious risk is controlled.

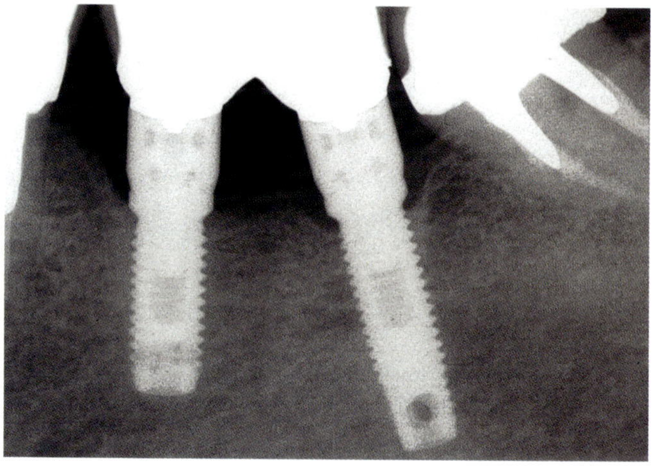

Fig 5-3n Implant-prosthetic rehabilitation in mandibular left quadrant. The third molar and first premolar are restored individually to predetermine occlusal guidance before implants are placed.

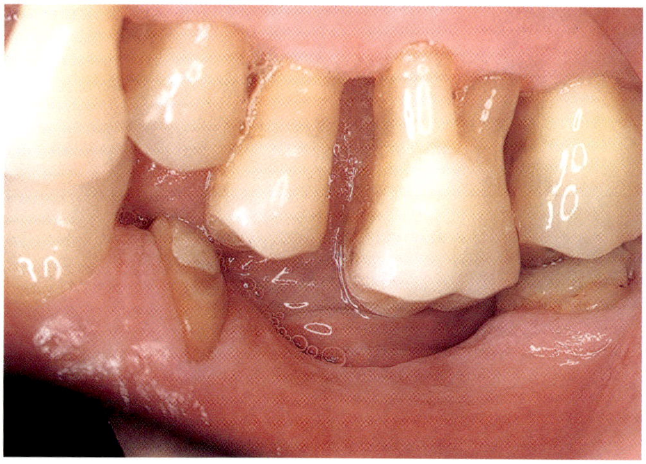

Fig 5-3o Before treatment.

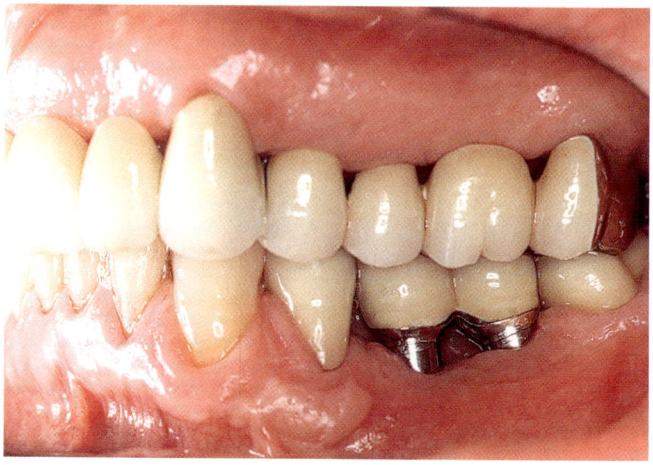

Fig 5-3p Periodontal-prosthetic rehabilitation is achieved. Local factors and risk sites have been eliminated. Risk for recurrence is controlled.

Aggressive Periodontitis

Aggressive periodontal diseases may present as several distinct disease subtypes occurring in otherwise healthy subjects. With aggressive periodontitis, there may be a hereditary component, and disease usually progresses rapidly. Aggressive periodontitis has been classified into two distinct subcategories: localized periodontitis and generalized periodontitis (American Academy of Periodontology 2000).

Moderate aggressive periodontitis

Clinical signs and symptoms

There is no direct correlation between the amount of bacterial deposit and severity of destruction. Likewise, disease progression is not linear, and attachment or bone loss may spontaneously accelerate or slow down.

Localized aggressive periodontitis (formerly known as juvenile periodontitis*)*

This periodontal disease is often associated with the presence of *Actinobacillus actinomycetemcomitans* and with neutrophil dysfunction. Onset generally occurs around puberty, and destruction is localized to permanent first molars and incisors. However, typical forms of the disease do exist. Serum analysis shows evidence of an intense primary antibody response to bacterial infection.

Generalized aggressive periodontitis (formerly known as rapidly progressing periodontitis*)*

This form of periodontal disease usually occurs in subjects younger than 30 years of age (Fig 5-4). Proximal attachment losses occur during periods of disease activity and involve at least three permanent teeth, other than the first molars and incisors. *A actinomycetemcomitans* and *Porphyromonas gingivalis* are frequently involved. There is also evidence of abnormal neutrophil function. However, antibody response has been shown to be weak.

Treatment goals and considerations

Treatment aims at attenuating or eliminating microbial etiologic factors as well as modifying predisposing risk factors. This helps in arresting disease progression and contributes to prevention of disease recurrence. Attachment regeneration may be attempted after favorable conditions have been established.

Management of aggressive periodontitis may be difficult or even impossible. This may be due to systemic factors, immune dysfunction, or a specific pathogenic flora.

Treatment methods are the same as those used for chronic forms of periodontitis. In some cases, however, the main treatment goal is simply to limit the rate of disease progression.

Medical screening is sometimes advised to rule out systemic disease; this is especially the case in younger patients presenting with advanced forms of periodontitis who respond poorly to periodontal treatment. In these cases, the periodontist should collaborate closely with the physician. This may modify some of the environmental risk factors.

Conventional mechanical treatment alone does not usually allow for satisfactory control of disease progression. Adjunct antimicrobial therapy eventually followed by surgery is therefore indicated. Long-term results depend on patient compliance and an appropriately scheduled supportive therapy regimen.

When deciduous teeth are involved, eruption of permanent teeth should be monitored to detect attachment loss. When there is evidence of familial predisposition to aggressive periodontitis, screening of other family members is recommended.

Conditions for success

Treatment of patients suffering from aggressive periodontitis (Fig 5-5) should aim at achieving the following goals:

- To reduce clinical signs of gingival inflammation (Fig 5-5d)
- To reduce probing depths (Fig 5-5e)
- To stabilize or gain clinical attachment (Fig 5-5f)
- To establish evidence of bone repair through radiographic evaluation (Fig 5-5h)
- To improve occlusal stability (see Fig 6-2)
- To reduce clinically detectable plaque to a level compatible with periodontal health

In some areas, these conditions may not be attained if:

- Gingival inflammation persists
- Periodontal pockets persist or aggravate
- There is progressive loss of clinical attachment
- Tooth mobility increases

Severity and risk factors

Risk factors for aggressive periodontitis include excessive buildup of bacterial plaque, presence of specific bacterial strains, a deleterious host response, tobacco use, and systemic disease. Severity is linked to these different parameters, but as with chronic periodontitis, locally aggravating factors (dental, periodontal, functional, or iatrogenic) are often involved.

Several factors may account for an altered host response:

- Neutrophil dysfunction
- HIV
- Smoking
- Diabetes
- Genetic predisposition
- Stress
- Hormonal imbalance
- Nutritional deficiency

Microbiologic perspective

The transition from periodontal health to aggressive periodontal disease is the consequence of a change in microbiologic balance:

- Change in total bacterial load
- Change in the beneficial/pathogenic bacterial ratio

Beneficial + + + / Pathogenic – ⇔ Beneficial – / **Pathogenic** + + +
Health **Disease**

The treatment goal is to modify the bacterial load–to–bacterial virulence ratio.

Histologic perspective

The passage from periodontal health to disease coincides with important tissue changes and cellular recruitments, all of which characterize the inflammatory state; however, these changes are reversible. Here again, there is a disturbance of the balance between elements involved in tissue destruction and those responsible for tissue repair. There is a gradual transition from one state to the other, and this transition should be considered in its temporal dimension when preparing a treatment plan.

It is important to remember that there is a delay between onset of the clinical signs of inflammation and those histologic disturbances that are responsible for them. Histologic changes (cellular, vascular) precede the appearance of clinical signs, such as redness, edema, bleeding, or production of gingival crevicular fluid. During the reversal of inflammation, on the other hand, clinical signs of gingival health are observed before a complete reversal of destructive processes occurs.

Inflammation – ⇔ **Inflammation** + + +
Health **Disease**

The treatment goal is to achieve conditions that promote tissue response.

As a general rule, the transition between health and disease is connected to the existence of risk factors, which are responsible for a homeostatic shift.

Risk factors – ⇔ **Risk factors** + + +
Health **Disease**

The treatment goal is to reduce or eliminate risk factors.

In conclusion

- There is no logic in using a sequential mechanical treatment quadrant after quadrant. Bacterial changes do occur in each quadrant, but there is a strong likelihood for renewed infection of one quadrant by another.
- Aggressive treatment under local anesthesia should be avoided because it may hinder cellular and tissue reorganization during tissue response and repair.
- Antibiotic therapy initiated too early in the course of treatment is a mistake and may induce a rebound effect. A primary reduction of bacterial load should be carried out before initiating massive antibiotic action. A progressive return to a favorable bacterial/host balance is preferable.
- Root scaling and planing in a single session, with or without antibiotic therapy, does not represent sufficient therapy for long-term periodontal stability.
- Root scaling and planing should be global and progressive and should take into account the patient's capacity to acquire adequate hygiene skills (see Fig 5-4).
- There is a greater risk for recurrence in aggressive periodontitis than in chronic periodontitis. Accordingly, periodontal maintenance should be more frequent, and bacterial analyses should be carried out when necessary.

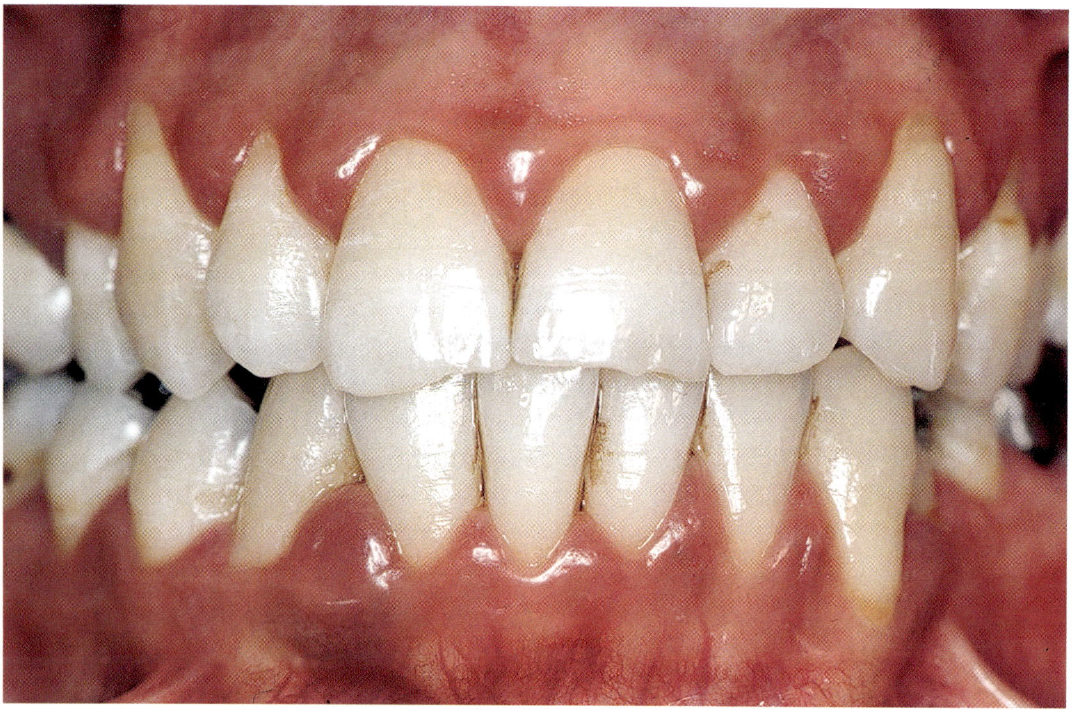

Fig 5-4a Generalized aggressive periodontitis in a 24-year-old male patient. Significant inflammation, small amounts of plaque deposits, and probing depths from 4 to 6 mm are seen. The patient smokes 15 cigarettes per day and reports a family history of periodontal disease. Pathogenic flora (*Tannerella forsythensis,* 5%) and commensal species (*Prevotella intermedia,* 30%, and *Fusobacterium nucleatum,* 10%) are present.

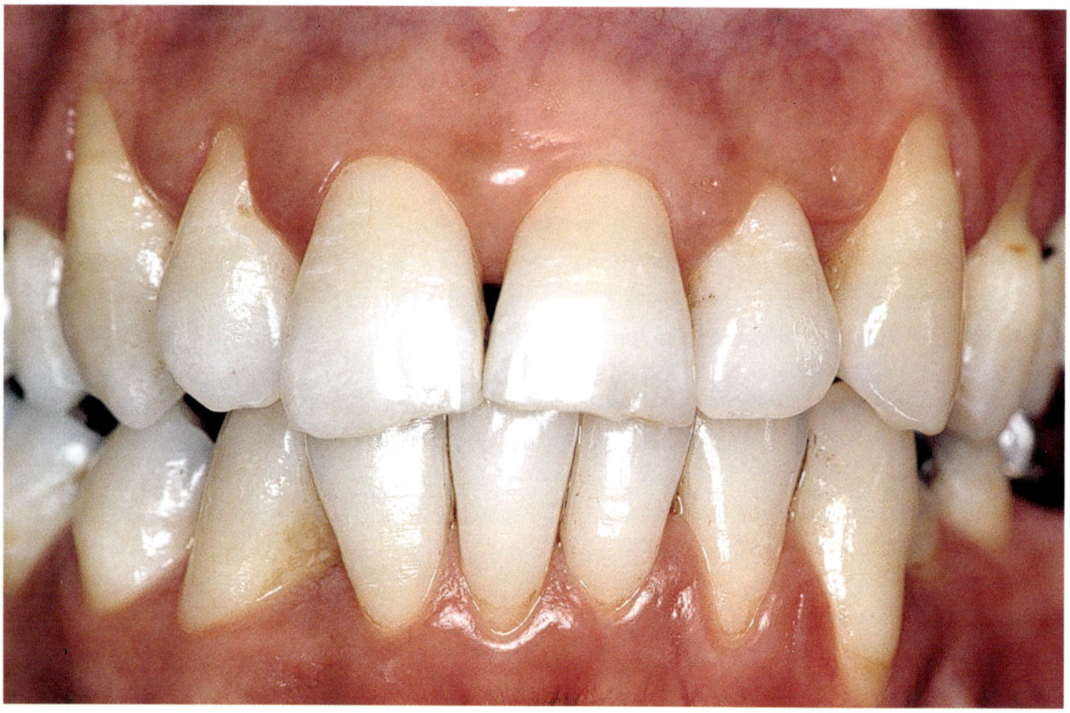

Fig 5-4b Treatment is as follows: oral hygiene instructions, reduction of smoking, removal of toothborne plaque and calculus (two sessions), and scaling and root planing (two sessions). At reevaluation, persistent bleeding in certain sites indicates the need for antimicrobial therapy with a 7-day course of metronidazole. Inflammation was completely reduced. Sites with pocket depths exceeding 4 mm underwent deep scaling and planing under local anesthesia.

Aggressive periodontitis and response potential

Aggressive periodontitis is characterized by rapid and irregularly distributed destruction. This disease subtype is characterized by a good response potential, especially when the predominant risk factor is bacterial. In advanced chronic periodontitis, this potential is expressed when local severity and complexity factors are corrected. The difficulty with this disease lies in understanding how to tailor appropriate treatment strategies: how exhaustive should treatment be in order to control risk and severity factors? Extraction decisions should not be made too early in treatment.

As a general rule, treatment of advanced chronic periodontitis (probing scores exceeding 6 mm) includes scaling and root planing performed in two consecutive phases, with or without antibiotic therapy. Treatment of aggressive periodontitis includes scaling and root planing performed in several consecutive phases, in addition to antibiotic therapy, which is administered before periodontal surgery is started.

Fig 5-5 Aggressive periodontitis with advanced attachment loss in a young adult.

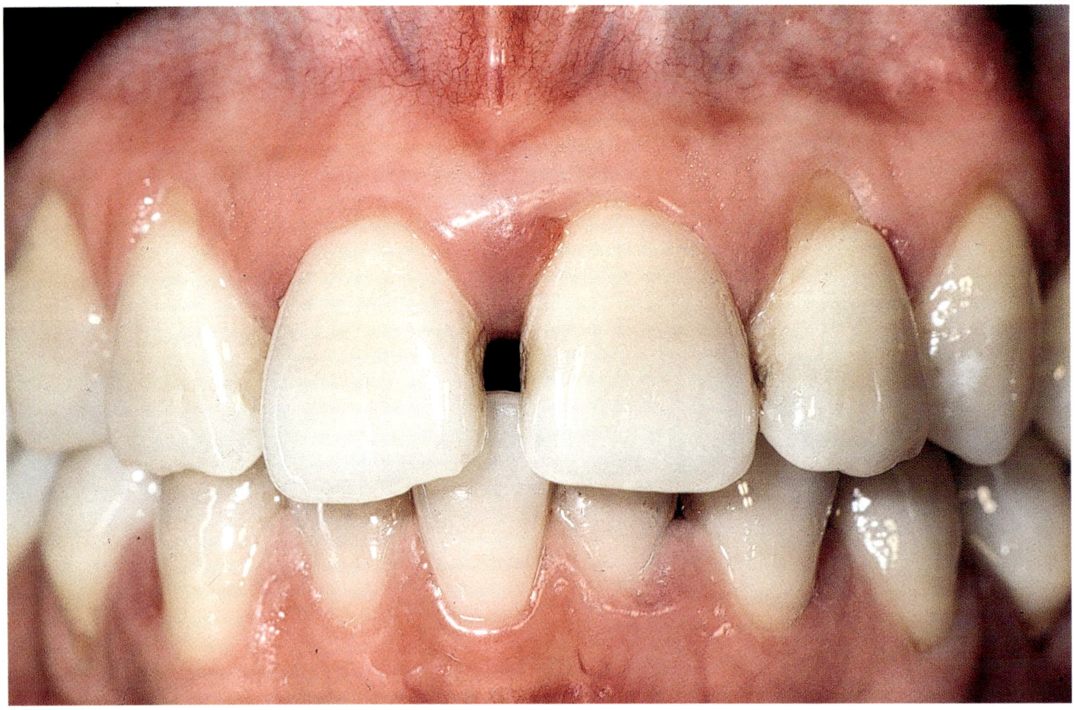

Fig 5-5a A 24-year-old, otherwise healthy, nonsmoking female patient who is mildly stressed. *Clinical signs:* Spontaneous bleeding, pain, mobility, migrations, recently developed diastema (within 6 months). Few plaque deposits and a mild degree of inflammation. *Risk factors:* Probable genetic predisposition. Deep pockets, if they persist after treatment, represent a risk for recurrence. *Diagnosis:* Moderate aggressive periodontitis with locally severe sites.

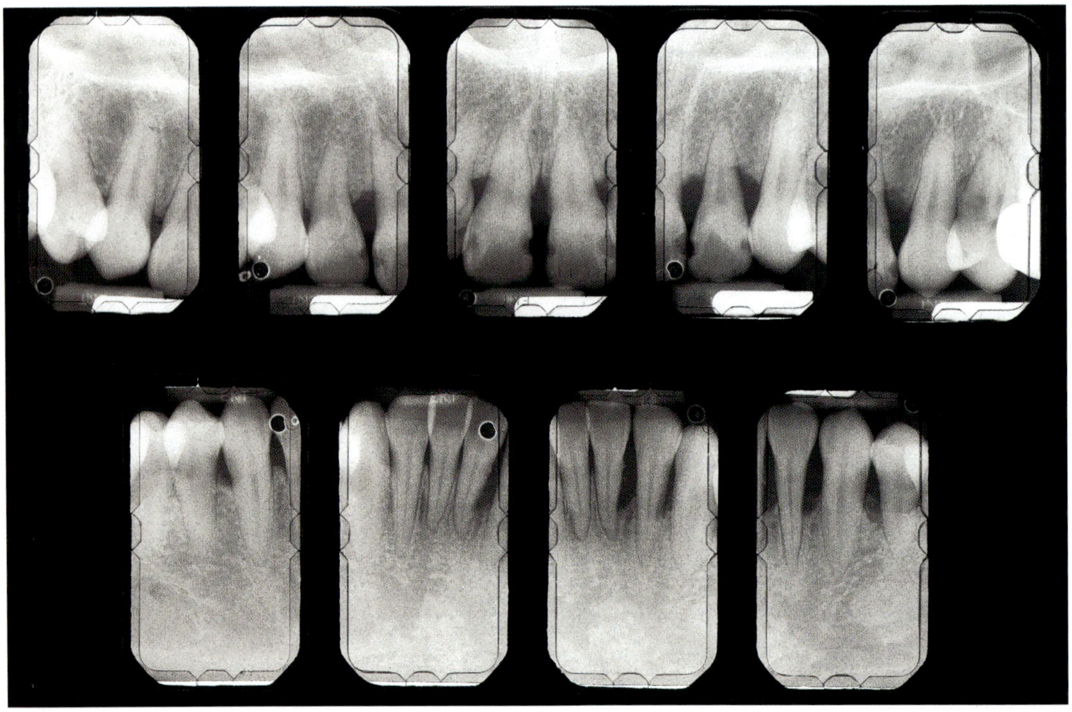

Fig 5-5b Generalized, irregular bone destruction (greater than 75% around the mandibular left central incisor), attachment loss, and pockets (4 to 6 mm around the mandibular left central incisor). *Severity factors:* Bacterial plaque and true infection, induced by exogenous pathogenic bacteria.

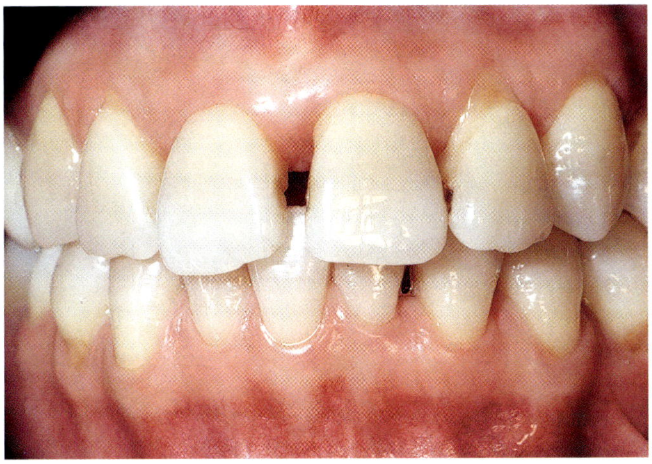

Fig 5-5c The first signs of inflammation appear after improvement of plaque control and initial cleaning sessions.

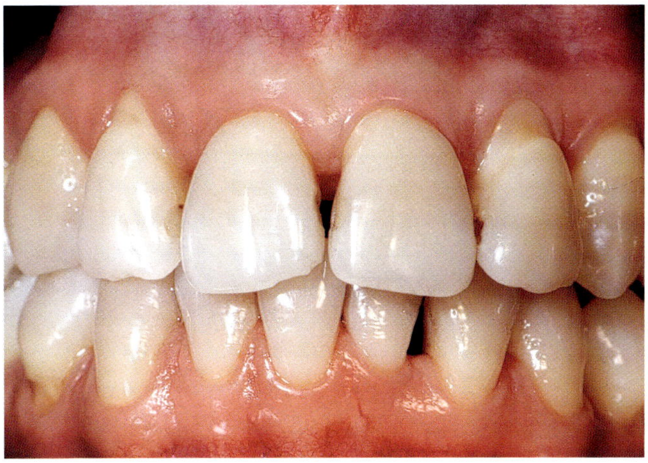

Fig 5-5d Etiologic treatment is performed: oral hygiene instructions, removal of toothborne plaque and calculus (one session), scaling and root planing (two sessions), antibiotic therapy (metronidazole 250 mg tid for 10 days), and periodontal surgery. Signs of inflammation disappear. Diastema closes spontaneously. Dental mobility is reduced as well.

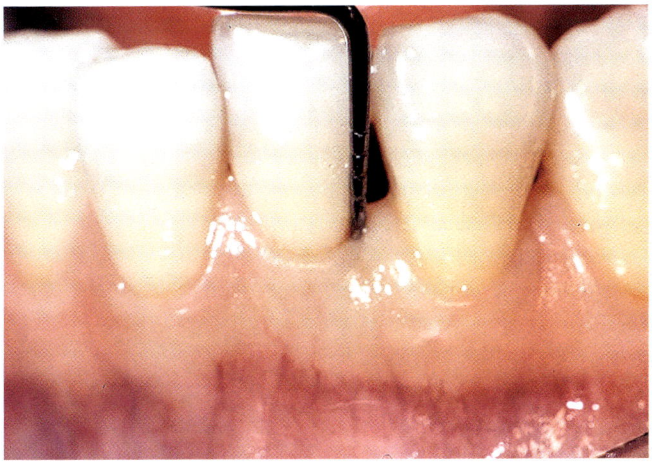

Fig 5-5e On the distal aspect of the mandibular left central incisor, the probing depth is 9 mm (attachment loss 7 mm).

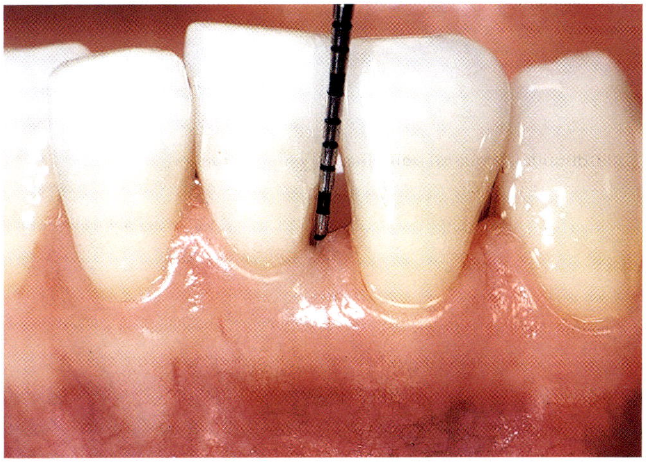

Fig 5-5f After treatment, the probing depth is 3 mm; pocket reduction is 6 mm, and attachment gain is 6 mm.

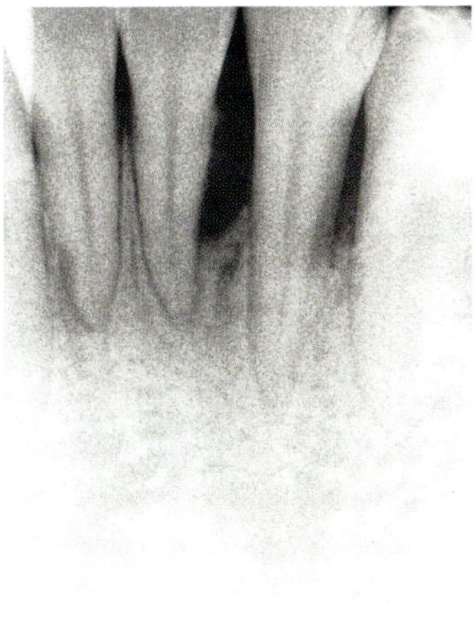

Fig 5-5g Bone destruction involves three-quarters of the root length.

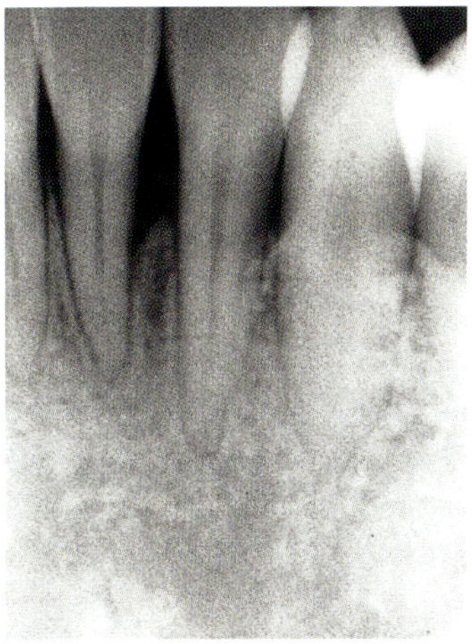

Fig 5-5h Bone repair is greater than 50%. All sites displaying attachment loss prior to treatment finally display attachment gains.

Response potential can be assessed through all signs of periodontal disease.

Adjunctive Therapy

6

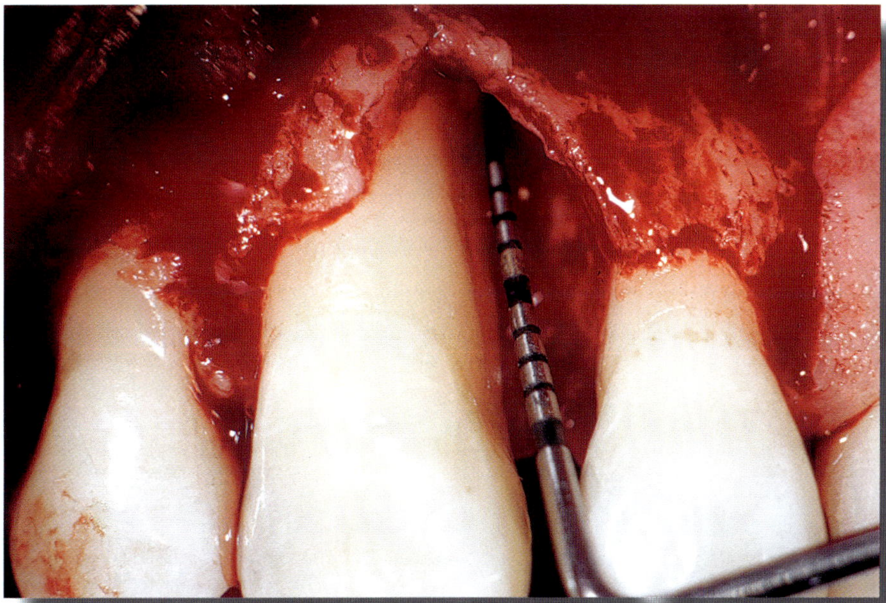

Aggressive Periodontitis and Occlusal Trauma

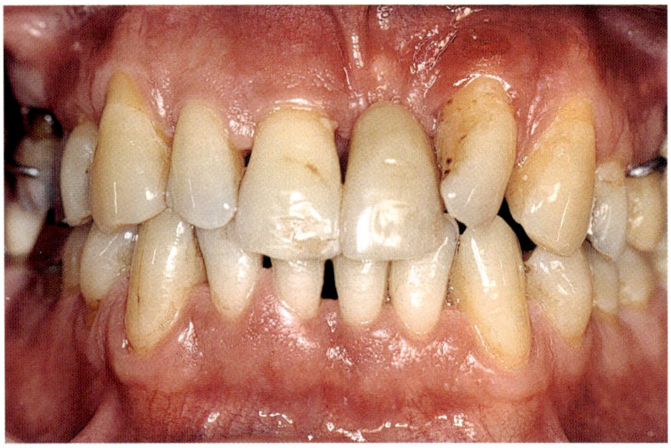

Fig 6-1a Aggressive periodontitis in a 50-year-old, otherwise healthy male patient experiencing stress at work. He is an occasional smoker. A partial denture replaces the missing maxillary left central incisor. Cultural analysis disclosed *Prevotella intermedia* (14.7%) and *Fusobacterium nucleatum* (2.4%). Infection type is commensal.

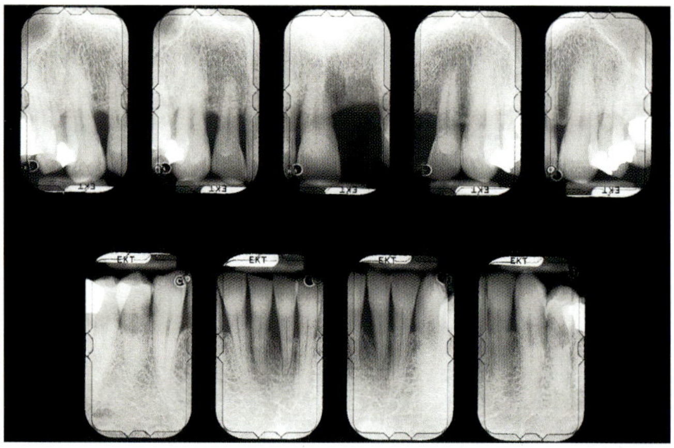

Fig 6-1b Bone destruction is irregularly distributed and is locally terminal around the maxillary right central and lateral incisors and is severe around the mandibular left central incisor. *Severity factors:* Significant plaque buildup; occlusal trauma induced by partial denture. *Risk factors:* Predisposition, stress.

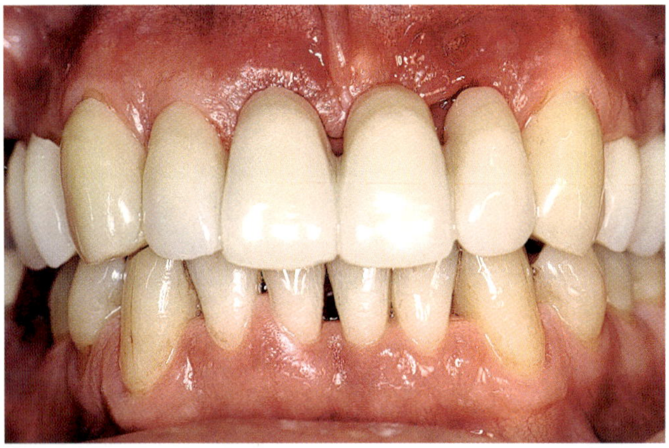

Fig 6-1c *Global treatment strategy:* Local treatment (removal of toothborne plaque, scaling and root planing), functional treatment (provisional crown and extraction of the maxillary right central incisor and left lateral incisor), occlusal rehabilitation (elimination of occlusal discrepancy on the mandibular left central incisor), antibiotic therapy (metronidazole 500 mg tid for 8 days), and periodontal surgery.

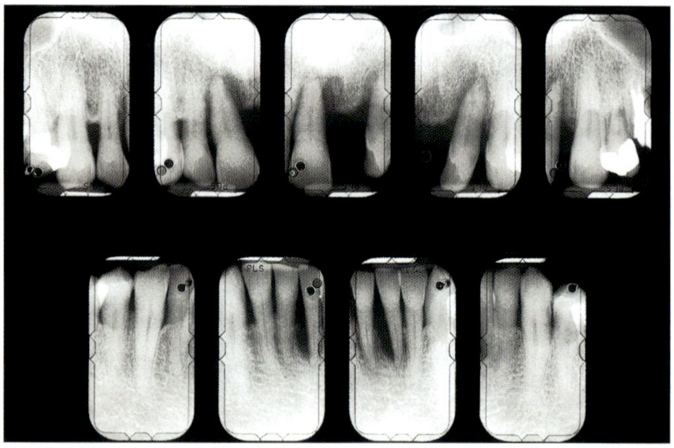

Fig 6-1d Endodontic treatment is carried out on the maxillary right canine and lateral incisor and the left canine to reduce the crown-root ratio. Note the significant repair occurring around the right lateral incisor and left canine.

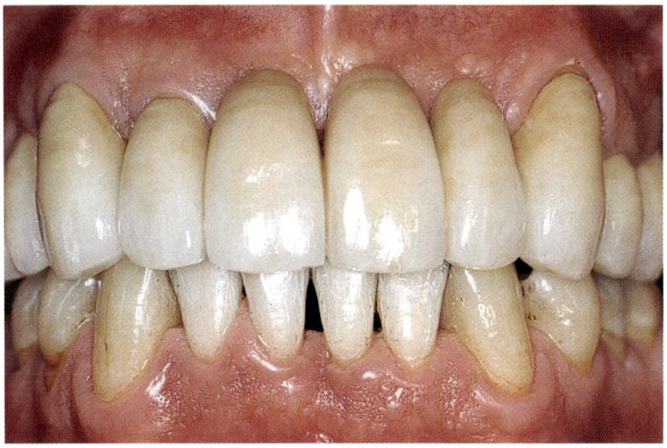

Fig 6-1e After prosthetic rehabilitation and supportive therapy three times a year, the patient is able to monitor accumulation of plaque.

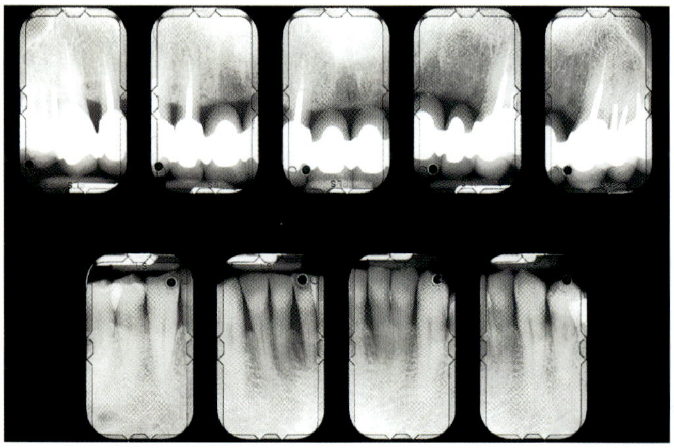

Fig 6-1f Favorable response potential (bone repair, attachment gain, reduction of pocket depth, and reduction of mobility) is easy to observe around the mandibular left central incisor.

Aggressive Periodontitis and Loss of Posterior Occlusal Support

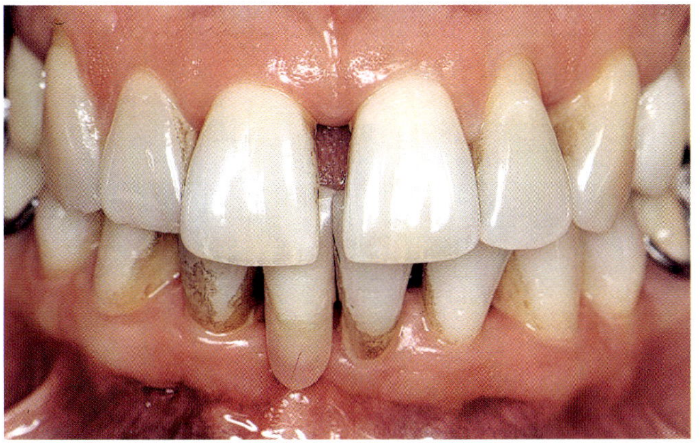

Fig 6-2a Aggressive periodontitis in a 49-year-old, otherwise healthy, nonsmoking female patient. *Clinical signs:* Few deposits, mild inflammatory signs, incisor migrations and egressions (newly onset diastema 1 year ago), mobility, pockets, no posterior contacts, functional disturbance, partial denture to replace the mandibular right central incisor. *Cultural analysis: P intermedia* (13.8%), *F nucleatum* (0.1%), *Capnocytophaga* spp (0.1%), *Campylobacter rectus* (0.1%); high plaque scores.

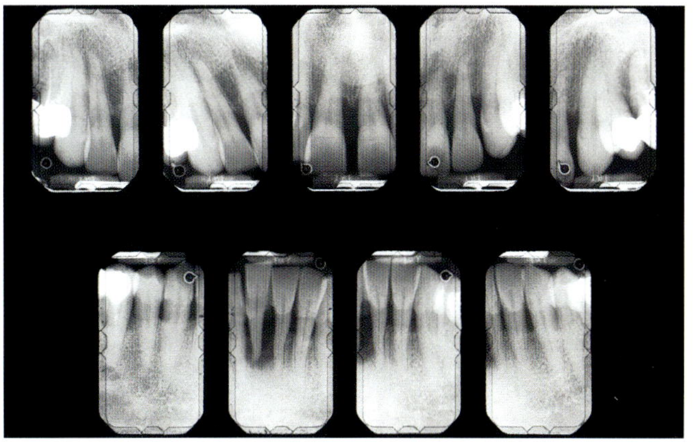

Fig 6-2b *Radiographic signs:* Significant, irregular bone destruction (terminal around the mandibular right central incisor before it was extracted). *Severity factors:* Local factors, functional factors (collapse of posterior occlusion). *Risk factors:* Possible predisposition. *Diagnosis:* Aggressive periodontitis involving infection by commensal flora.

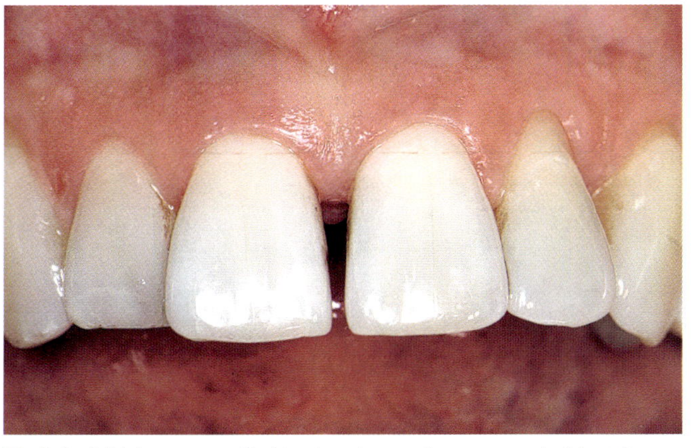

Fig 6-2c *Initial treatment:* Oral hygiene instructions, removal of dental plaque and calculus, provisional occlusofunctional rehabilitation and restoration of lateral occlusion, scaling and root debridement. Clinical signs indicate improvement: the diastema is narrowing.

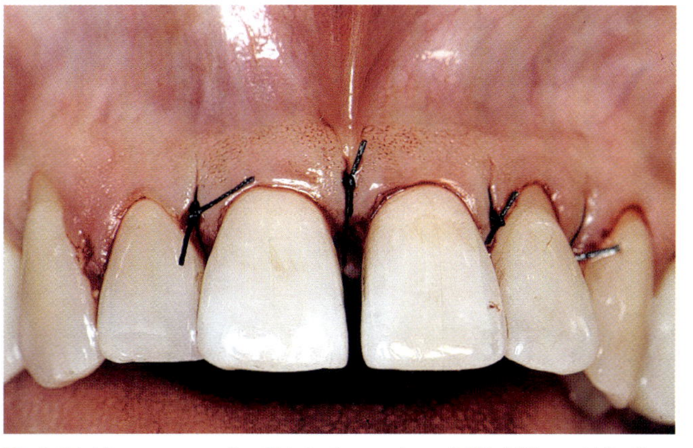

Fig 6-2d After a course of antibiotic therapy (amoxicillin 500 mg tid for 8 days), undertaken because of persistent bleeding in deep pockets, surgery is performed in areas where persistent pockets display probing depths exceeding 5 mm.

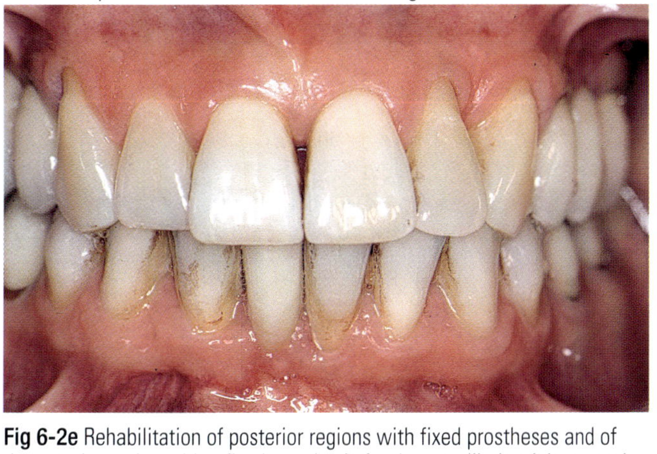

Fig 6-2e Rehabilitation of posterior regions with fixed prostheses and of the anterior region with a fixed prosthesis for the mandibular right central incisor) is performed. The diastema reduced spontaneously after surgery.

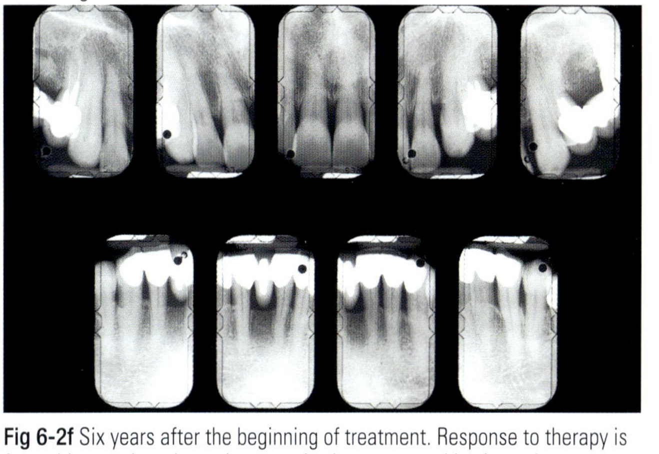

Fig 6-2f Six years after the beginning of treatment. Response to therapy is favorable: repair and attachment gains have occurred in sites where destruction was most significant.

Advanced Chronic Periodontitis with Multiple Associated Disorders

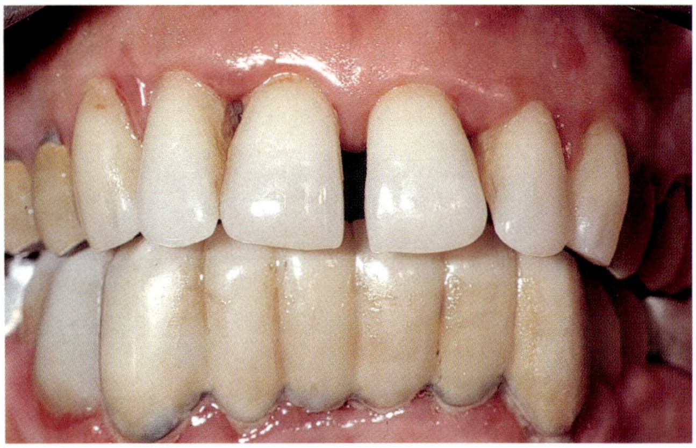

Fig 6-3a A 55-year-old, otherwise healthy, nonsmoking female patient. The patient has never undergone any dental cleanings and brushes once a day. *Signs:* Deposits, presence of plaque, severe inflammation, halitosis, occlusal disturbance, anterior overjet, diastema, mobility, discomfort, and pain. *Multiple local factors:* Bacterial, dental, prosthetic, and functional. *Diagnosis:* Advanced chronic periodontitis.

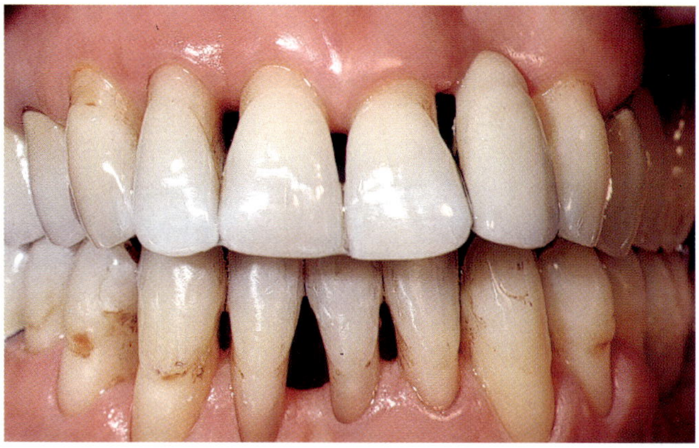

Fig 6-3b Treatment consists of managing inflammation and correcting local and functional factors. Periodontal surgery is performed throughout the dentition. Three sites receive specific treatment: the maxillary left lateral incisor and mandibular right central incisor were extracted, and the maxillary left canine underwent guided tissue regeneration therapy (see Figs 6-5a to 6-5h).

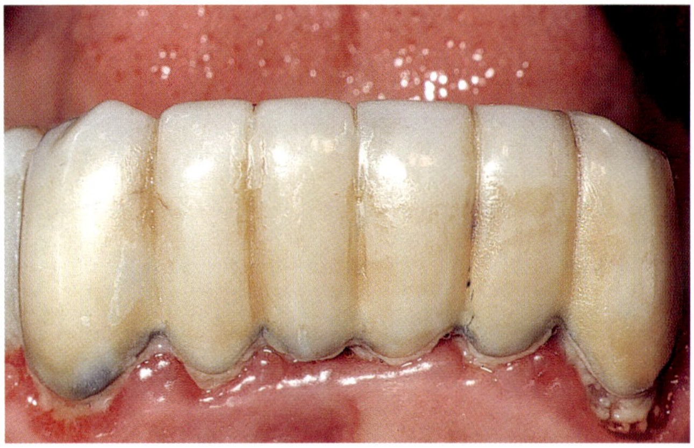

Fig 6-3c The goal of this iatrogenic prosthetic device was to correct a primary anterior underbite and to act as a splinting device for the incisors. A new underbite appeared, most likely secondarily to lingual hyperfunction.

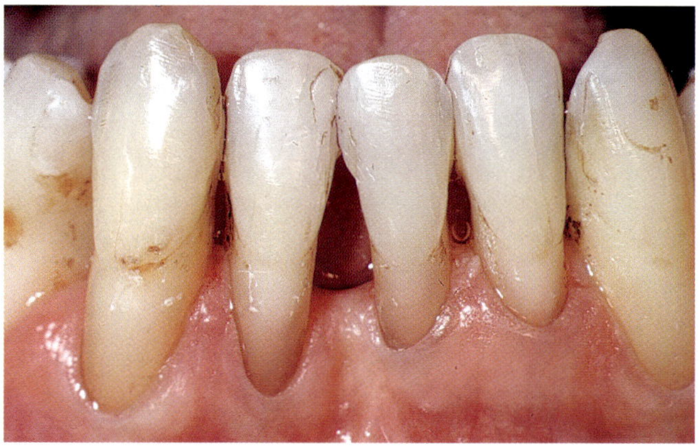

Fig 6-3d When the anterior prosthetic device is removed, the incisors are intact. The right central incisor is extracted. This promotes spontaneous realignment of the three remaining incisors, correction of ectopic buccal position of the mandibular right canine, and spontaneous closure of the diastema between the maxillary central incisors, all of which contribute to restoring periodontal health.

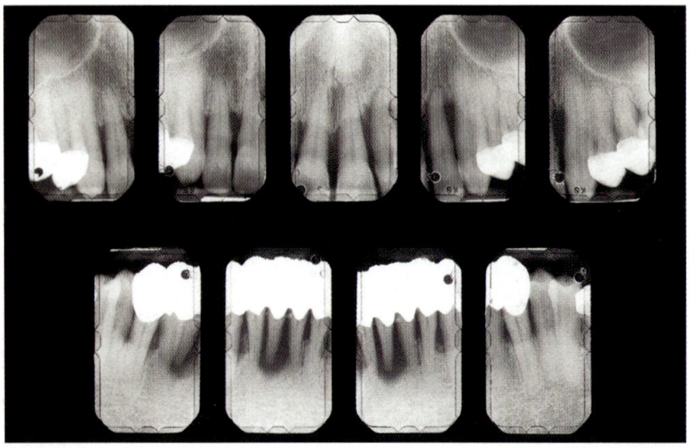

Fig 6-3e Destruction around anterior teeth is extremely severe (particularly around the maxillary left lateral incisor and canine, the mandibular central incisors, and the right lateral incisor). Attachment losses and pocket depths are very significant. A conservative approach allows for a continuous evaluation of the response to treatment.

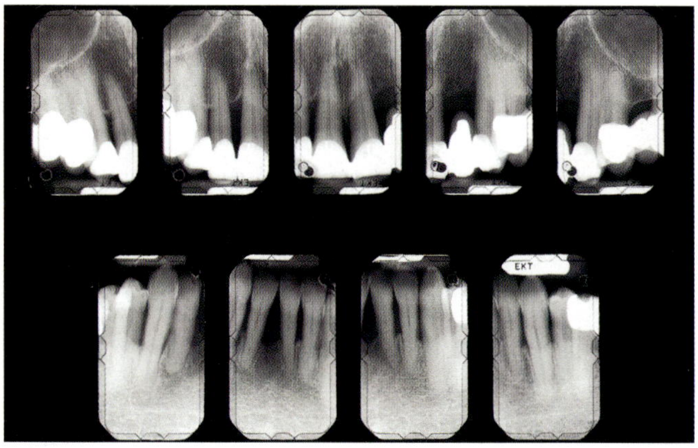

Fig 6-3f After treatment, the extent of repair can be appreciated throughout the periodontal tissue, as can the significant tissue regeneration that has occurred on the mesial aspect of the maxillary left canine (see Figs 6-5a to 6-5h).

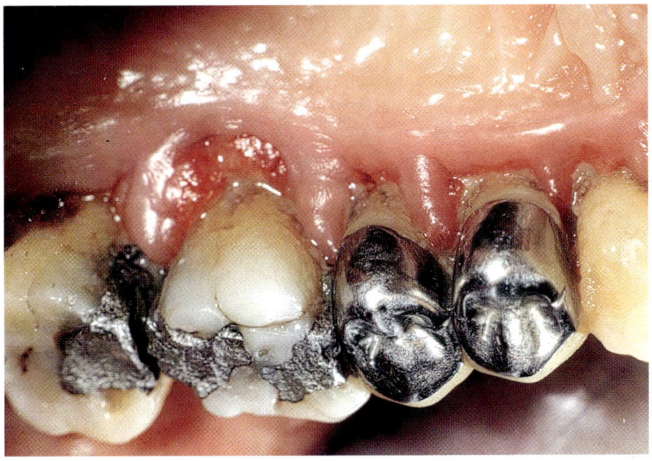

Fig 6-3g On the palatal aspects, signs of inflammation are extensive. They are correlated with exceptional amounts of plaque found in their vicinity. The first molar presents a longitudinal fissure and cannot be preserved.

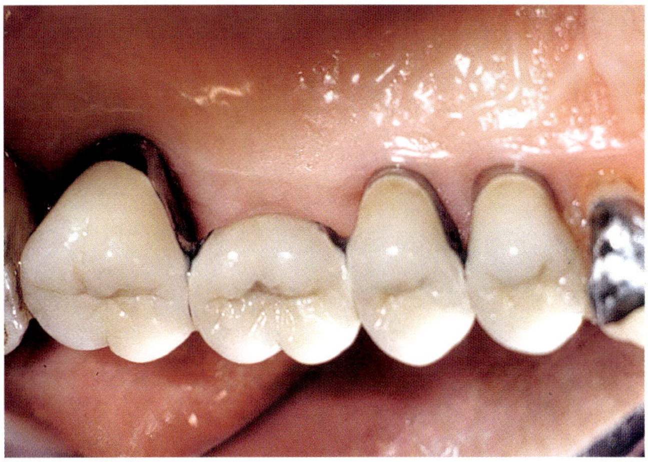

Fig 6-3h Favorable response to periodontal treatment, which consisted of local and surgical management. Antibiotic therapy (amoxicillin 500 tid for 8 days) is administered during the days before and after regeneration surgery around the maxillary left canine.

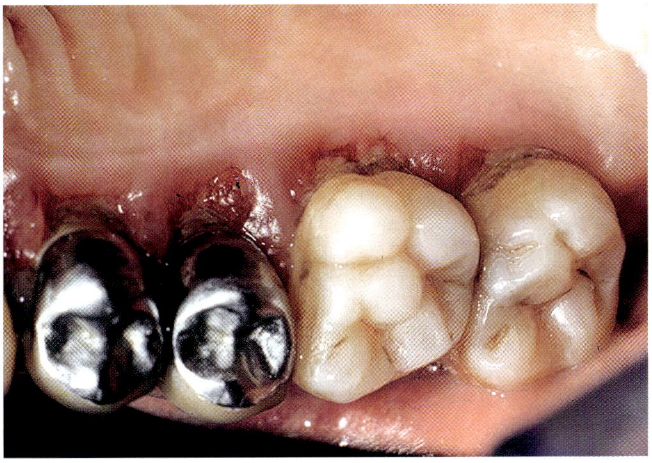

Fig 6-3i Inflammation is more severe in sites where restorations are poorly adapted.

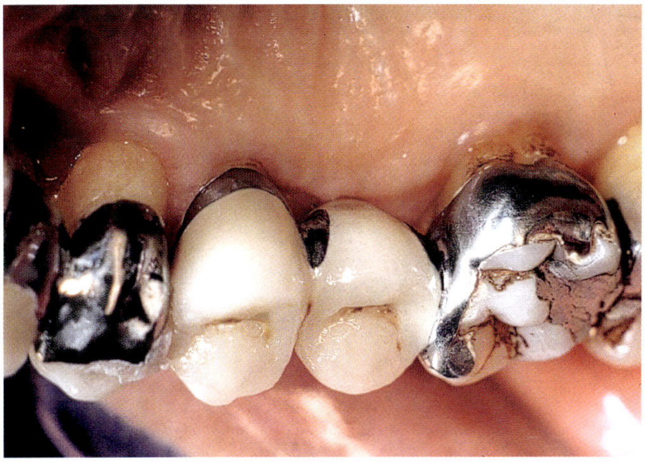

Fig 6-3j The second premolar had exhibited terminal bone destruction and Class IV mobility and was extracted. Favorable periodontal response occurred following treatment. Abutment design on the molar allows for future access to pulp in the event that root amputation is indicated (Class II).

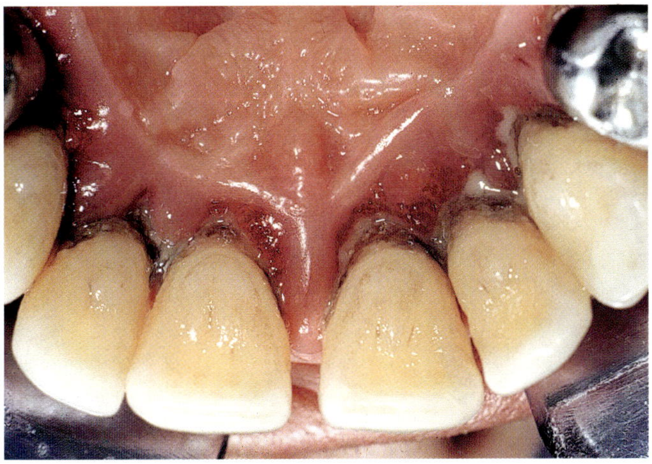

Fig 6-3k There is a direct relation between the degree of inflammation and the amount of plaque-derived biofilm.

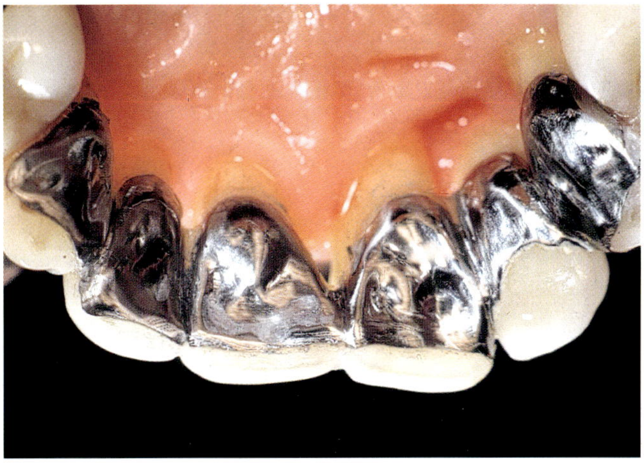

Fig 6-3l A bonded, removable pontic-splint replaces the left lateral incisor, stabilizes the central incisors, and ensures splinting before guided tissue regeneration is initiated around the left canine.

Advanced Chronic Periodontitis and Orthodontics

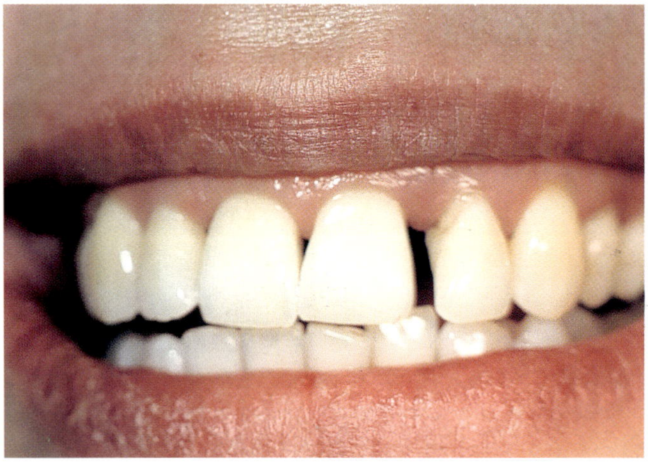

Fig 6-4a Advanced chronic periodontitis in a 45-year-old female patient. Dental displacements and secondary diastemata are significant. There is no canine guidance on the left. The maxillary left lateral incisor presents Class III mobility. Esthetics are compromised.

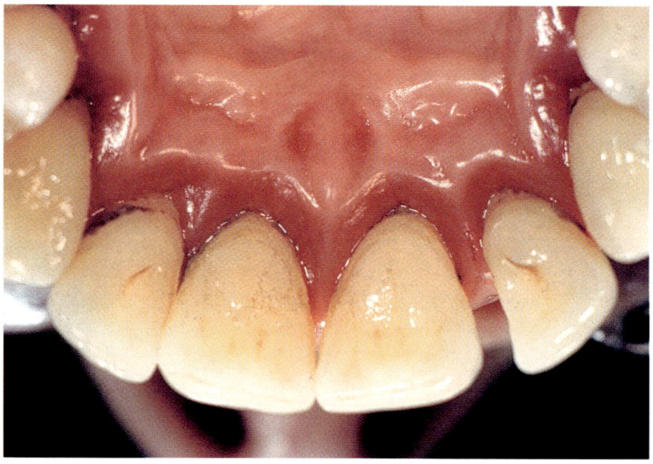

Fig 6-4b Signs of inflammation are generalized and correlate to the amount of bacterial deposits. Infection is commensal.

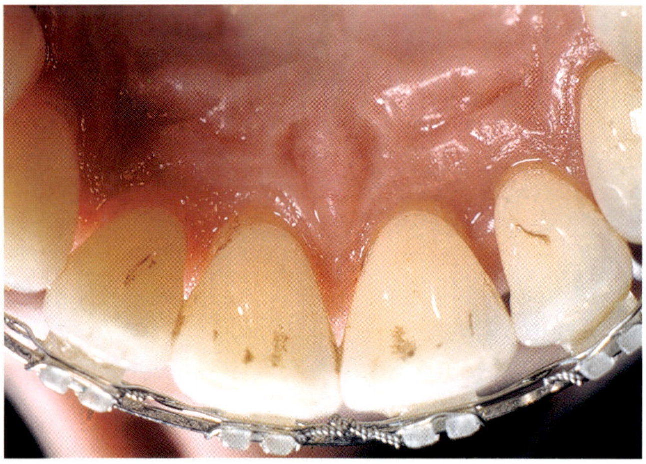

Fig 6-4c Infection control is achieved through the usual protocol: crown and root debridement, scaling, and root planing (four sessions), followed by periodontal surgery. Because teeth malpositions have not improved, orthodontic management is required.

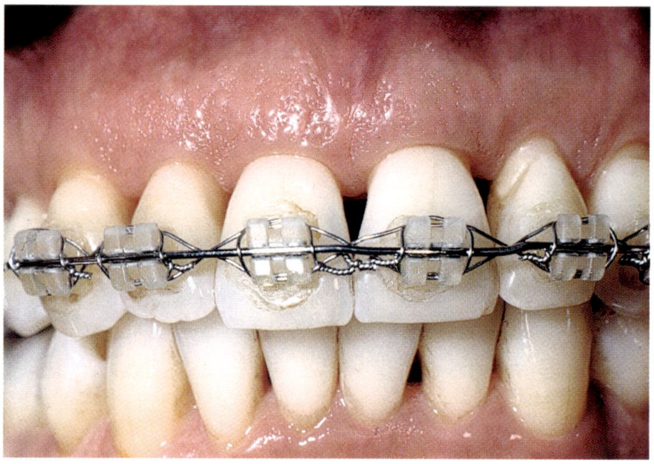

Fig 6-4d Dental displacements and diastemata have been corrected. Note healthy gingival tissue.

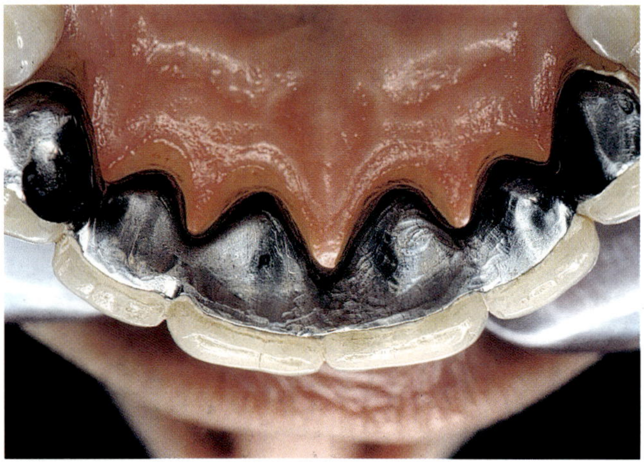

Fig 6-4e A bonded splint stabilizes the anterior teeth, canine to canine.

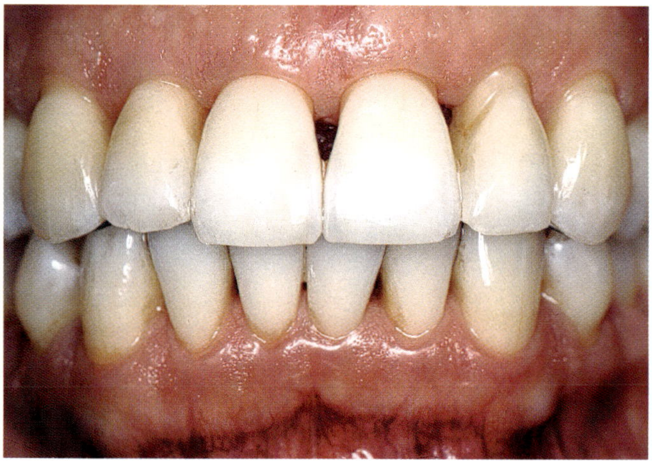

Fig 6-4f Periodontal health, function, and esthetics are restored.

High-Risk Sites

Areas of destruction most often display an uneven distribution in advanced periodontitis. Sites associated with higher risk for recurrence are those areas exhibiting poor response to periodontal surgery, even though overall improvement may have occurred. These sites become potential reservoirs for pathogenic bacteria. Subgingival recolonization from these sites increases the chances for disease recurrence or progression. In addition, plaque control cannot be carried out appropriately and durably in these sites. Finally, when the balance between pathogenic and beneficial bacteria is unfavorable, these sites continue to undergo attachment loss. Adequate adjunctive treatment should be initiated. There are three distinct types of risk sites:

- Deep pockets
- Interradicular lesions
- Mobile teeth

Deep pockets and bone defects

Before initiating any specific treatment in a given site, the severity and complexity factors mentioned earlier should be corrected. Pocket depth reduction occurs after initial treatment of inflammation is completed and as a consequence of ensuing reparative tissue response:

- *Gingival retraction + attachment gain = pocket reduction* (in the case of a supraosseous pocket). Remember that when probing inflamed tissue, the extremity of the probe penetrates the connective attachment tissue, well beyond the epithelial attachment. In contrast, the epithelial connective tissue of healthy periodontal tissue is able to withstand probing. Probing should not be performed too early in treatment.
- *Gingival retraction + attachment gain + bone gain = pocket reduction* (see Fig 5-5).

Assessment of these clinical parameters is necessary to evaluate treatment efficacy, response to treatment, and whether adjunct therapy is indicated.

Bone defects

Residual deep pockets are usually associated with the presence of bony lesions that have responded poorly to initial therapy. Specific adjunctive therapy consists of carrying out reparative surgery through guided tissue regeneration or bone grafting. Numerous different grafting materials have been assessed in clinical studies: these include autogenous graft tissues, decalcified and calcified allografts, xenografts (purified bovine-derived calcified bone matrix or porcine-derived enamel matrix components), and alloplastic bone substitutes (synthetic hydroxyapatite, tricalcic phosphates, and bioactive ceramic materials). Most of these materials serve as guides for the regeneration of bone tissue. Some of them, including growth factors, actually elicit bone regeneration, though their clinical applications need further evaluation.

The goal of periodontal regenerative techniques is the restoration of connective attachment tissue and enhancement of the growth of new cementum tissue, periodontal ligament, and bone tissues (Fig 6-5).

Regeneration of interproximal bone defects can only be performed through guided tissue regeneration, using resorbable or nonresorbable membranes, which are synthetic or animal-derived. Results are difficult to predict. Membranes are frequently distorted, particularly in large lesions; this reduces the regeneration rate. In addition, when the membrane is exposed, it is highly susceptible to colonization by plaque; this delays proper healing and may compromise the overall outcome.

A frequent cause for failure in restorative periodontal therapy is premature use of regenerative techniques during the course of treatment, especially before adequate infection control has been achieved (Nowzari and Slots 1994). First-line conditions for tissue healing need to be created. The morphology of existing lesions is a crucial factor in predicting the outcome.

Prognosis is better for deep, narrow lesions than for shallow, wide lesions such as osseous craters.

Nowadays, a wide array of periodontal techniques has rendered complete periodontal regeneration a realistic objective. These techniques include grafting (space occupied by a substitute), guided tissue regeneration (blood clot protection, barrier effect), and stimulation of osteogenesis.

Composite graft materials such as those associating autogenous bone or calcified bone tissues (Bio-Oss, Osteohealth) with a double collagen membrane (Bio-Gide, Osteohealth) were used in humans and studied by Camelo et al (2000), who reported satisfactory results (Fig 6-6).

Clinical, radiographic, and histologic outcomes were as follows:

- At 9 months postoperative, all clinical parameters were improved, with pocket depth reduction, attachment gain, and bone grafting.
- Histologic examination revealed the presence of newly formed cementum tissue with collagen-fiber insertions, as well as newly formed bone tissue at the surface of both types of graft particles. The mean length of the new attachment was found to be 4.33 mm.

Suggested protocol for regenerative techniques:

- Scaling and root planing
- Full width flap + curettage + root planing
- Root demineralization and decontamination with tetracycline
- Autogenous cancellous bone obtained from donor site
- Autogenous bone plus Bio-Oss mix for defect filling
- Cover site with Bio-Gide plus primary suture
- Postoperative antiobiotic therapy with chlorhexidine mouthwashes for 8 weeks
- Follow-up examination and supragingival cleaning at 7, 14, and 21 days postoperative. Oral hygiene recommendations. Supragingival removal of toothborne plaque at 4, 6, and 8 weeks, then every month until biopsy at 9 months postoperative (Camelo et al 2001).

Guided tissue regeneration for treatment of an osseous lesion

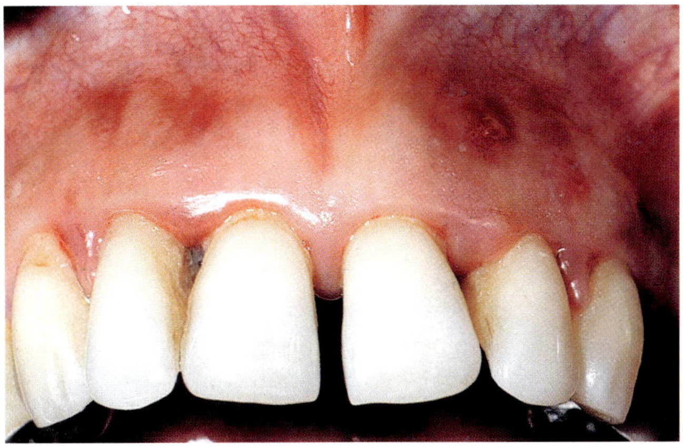

Fig 6-5a Patient with advanced chronic periodontitis seen in Fig 6-3.

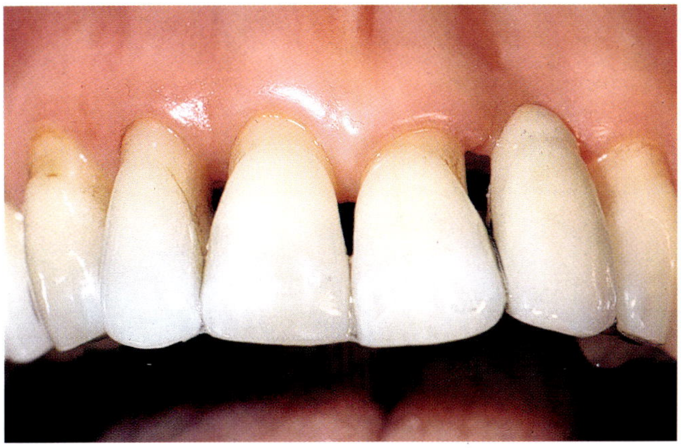

Fig 6-5b Treatment of periodontitis has been concluded. A splint adapts to the anterior teeth, and a prosthesis replaces the left lateral incisor, which was previously extracted.

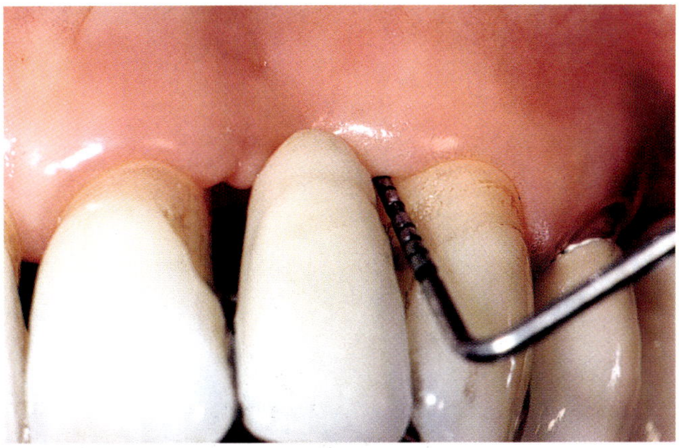

Fig 6-5c Probing depth on the mesial aspect of the canine is 10 mm. To provide access to the site, the prosthetic element replacing the left lateral incisor can be removed from its base.

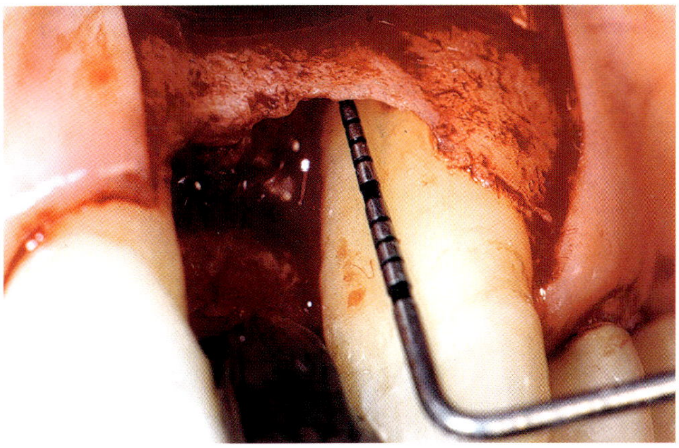

Fig 6-5d Attachment loss is evaluated at 13 mm. After lesion curettage, the root surface is meticulously prepared. The periodontal ligament space is then carefully opened. This promotes bleeding and clot formation.

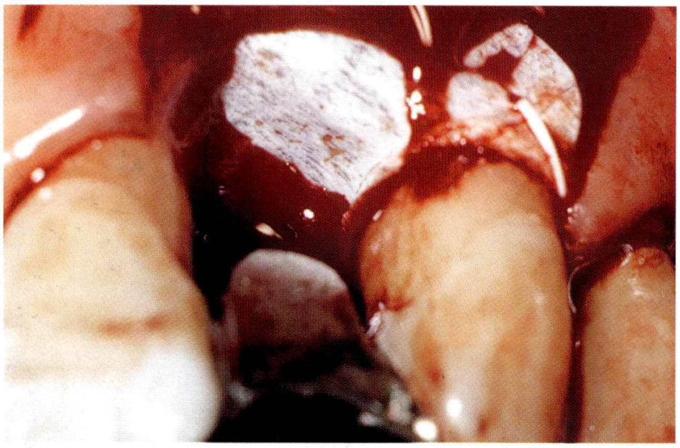

Fig 6-5e A nonresorbable membrane is fitted and tightly adapted around the tooth. The flap is then sutured to close off the surgical site. The healing phase is the most crucial. No plaque should be allowed to develop in the surgical area.

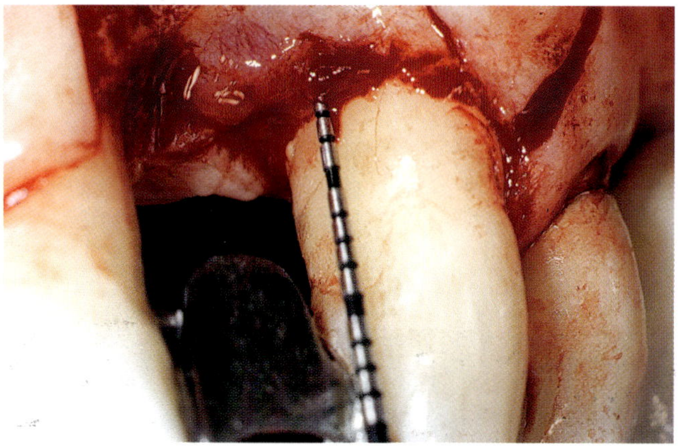

Fig 6-5f The membrane is removed 6 weeks after surgery. A firm, raspberry-red tissue is visible and adheres to the root surface. More than 8 mm of periodontal attachment has been restored.

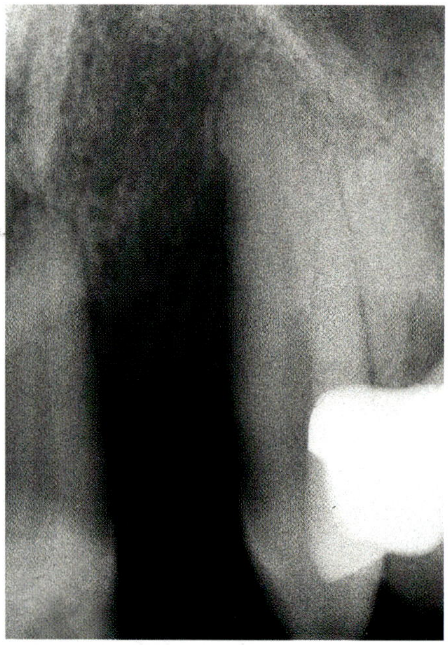

Fig 6-5g Radiograph of the lesion before guided tissue regeneration.

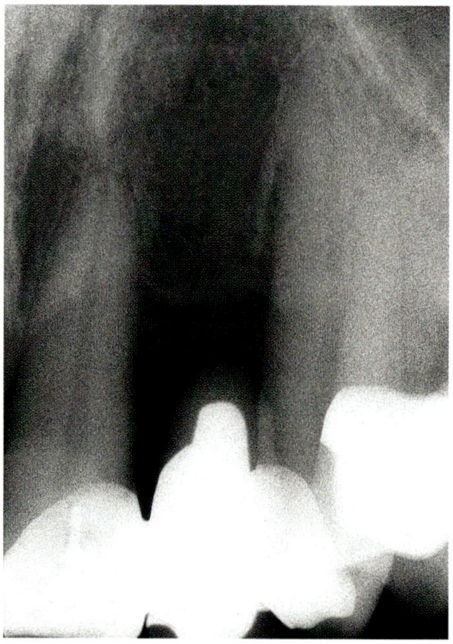

Fig 6-5h Bone regeneration 4 years later matches attachment gain recorded when the membrane was removed.

Treatment of an osseous lesion with bone grafting and regeneration

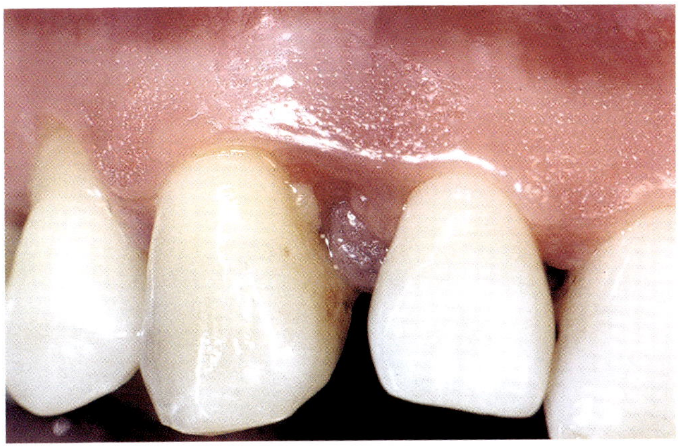

Fig 6-6a Aggressive periodontitis in a 45-year-old female patient with *Porphyromonas gingivalis* infection and trauma (nibbling parafunctional habit on the canine).

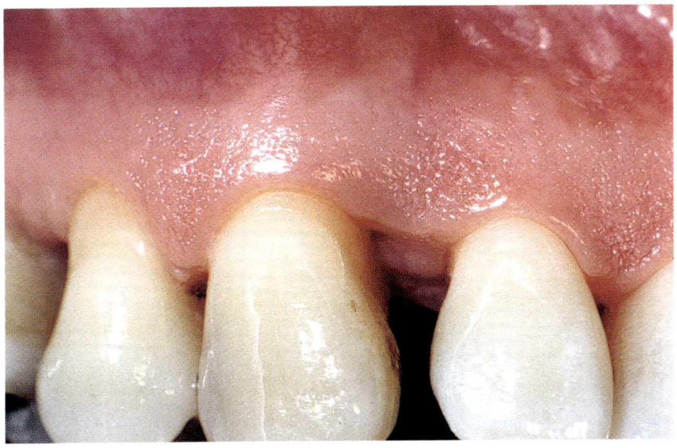

Fig 6-6b After global therapy, a periodontal pocket persists around the maxillary right central incisor.

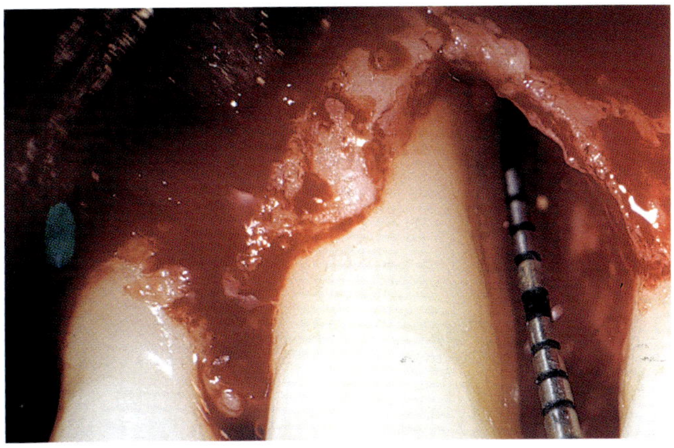

Fig 6-6c Attachment loss is estimated at 14 mm. Scaling and root planing are performed. A 1-minute application of tetracycline (tetracycline hydrochloride plus saline) on the root surface improves surface preparation.

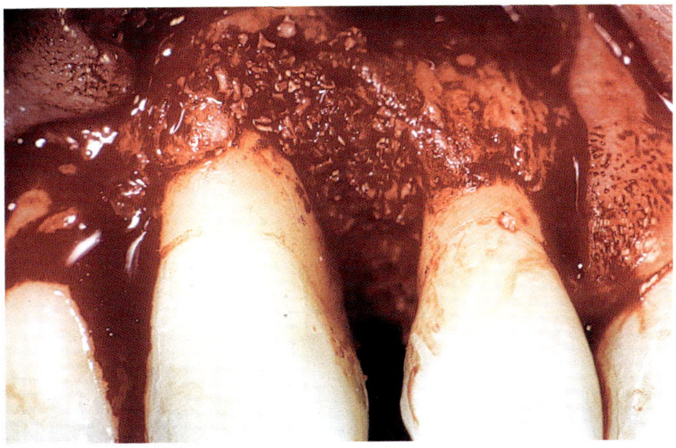

Fig 6-6d Particles of Bio-Oss mixed into the blood clot form a firm coagulum that can be fitted to replace the destroyed septum. A resorbable Bio-Gide membrane then covers the site. The flap is closed hermetically as much as possible. A surgical dressing is placed, and prophylactic antibiotic therapy and local antiseptic measures are prescribed.

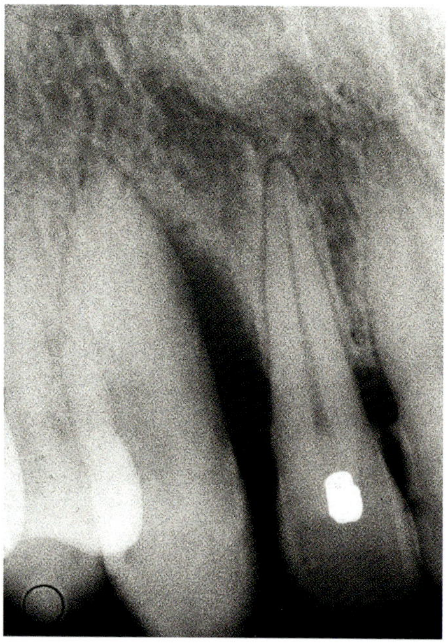

Fig 6-6e Bone destruction reaches the periapical region.

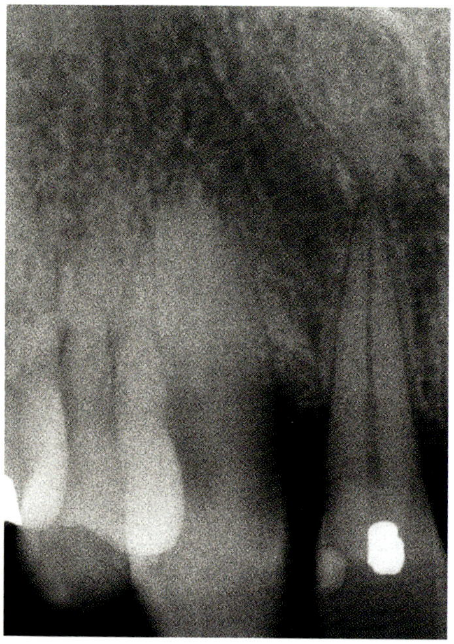

Fig 6-6f Outcome of the grafting procedure, 3 years after surgery. True regeneration can be expected with this technique.

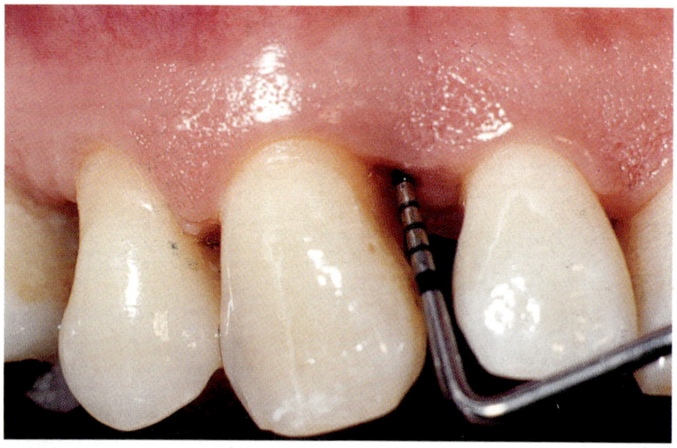

Fig 6-6g Recorded pocket depth is 11 mm preoperatively.

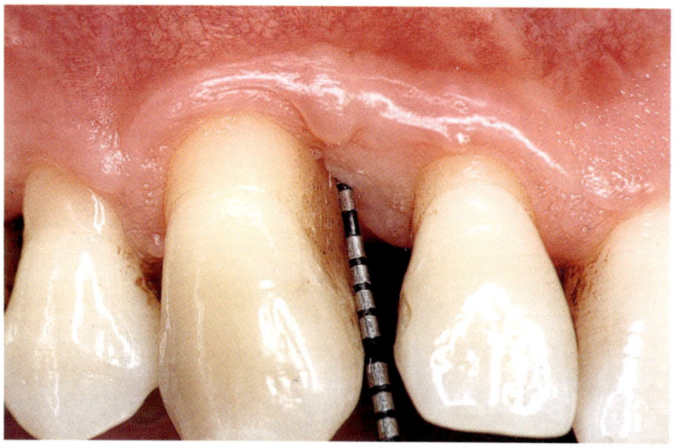

Fig 6-6h Three years after surgery, periodontal tissue is healthy. Pocket depth reduction and attachment gain are evaluated at 9 mm.

Interradicular lesions and conservative treatment

In Class I furcations, horizontal bone loss is less than one third of the tooth width; Class II lesions feature horizontal bone loss more than one third of the root width; Class III lesions feature through-and-through bone loss. Treatment should aim at promoting proper elimination of plaque and bacterial biofilm, as well as preparing dental and periodontal anatomies that are compatible with hygiene measures.

> When periodontal supportive therapy is performed scrupulously, a conservative approach to molars presenting furcation involvement is ideal (Fig 6-7). Statistically, success rates at 10 years postoperative are high (greater than 80%) (Svårdström and Wennström 2000).

Use of scaling and root planing alone does not allow for complete biofilm elimination in these sites, especially when probing depths are significant. These lesions therefore require closer attention than those found in the vicinity of single-rooted teeth. Optimal elimination of calculus is possible when surgery and scaling and root planing are associated in two consecutive operative steps. Also, pathogenic bacteria may be effectively and durably eradicated after subtractive bone surgery. Subsequent use of regenerative techniques is possible, though the outcome is often difficult to predict. The outcome is often disappointing for Class III furcation lesions. Amputation and resection techniques have progressively been set aside with the growing use of implant technology (Fig 6-8).

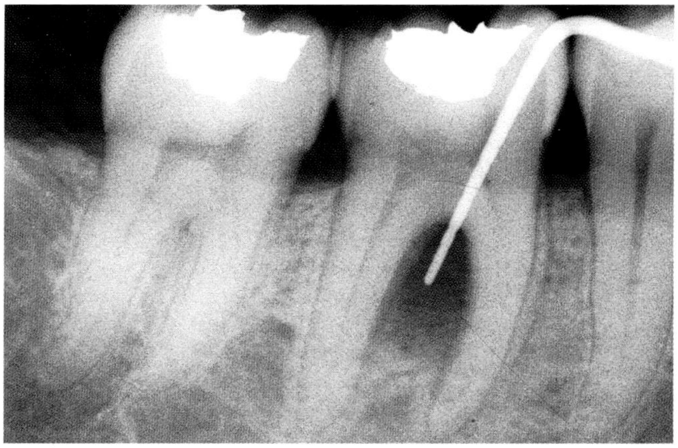

Fig 6-7a Localized advanced periodontitis featuring a Class III lesion. Grafting with nonresorbable porous hydroxyapatite was performed in 1985.

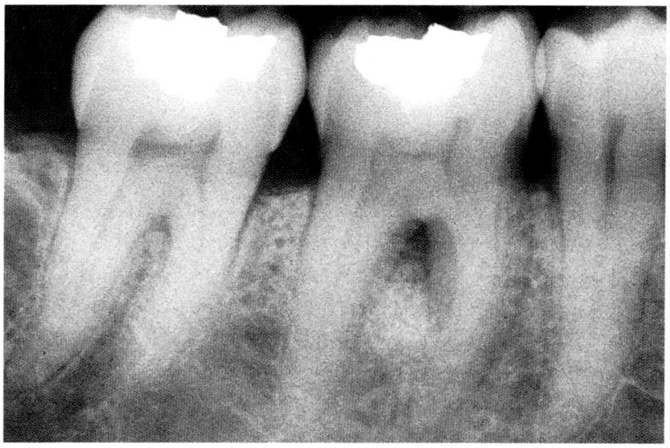

Fig 6-7b The tooth is still functional 14 years later, and periodontal health is well maintained. Periodontal maintenance has been performed three times a year.

Interradicular lesions and implants

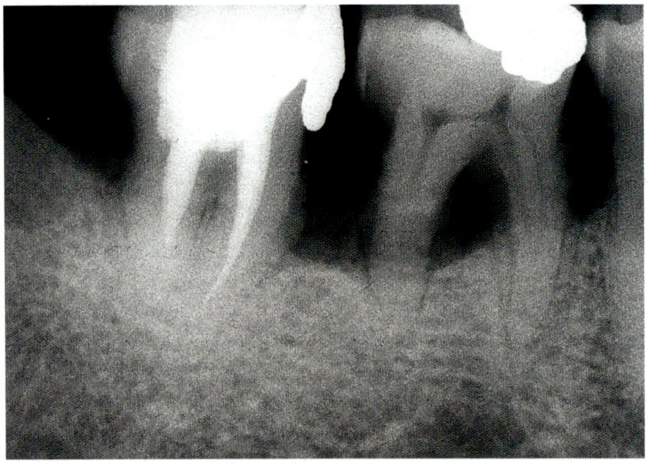

Fig 6-8a Advanced chronic periodontitis in a 45-year-old male with Class III lesion on the first molar and a Class I lesion on the second molar.

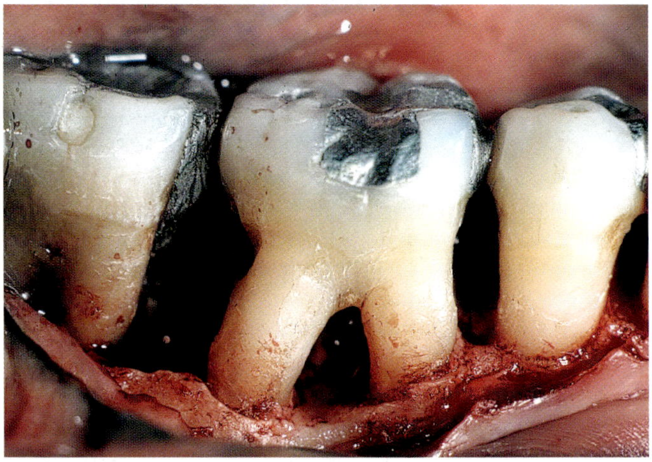

Fig 6-8b Surgical therapy, performed in 1983, consisted of an apically positioned flap with ostectomy to reduce bony craters. Periodontal maintenance therapy was performed twice a year.

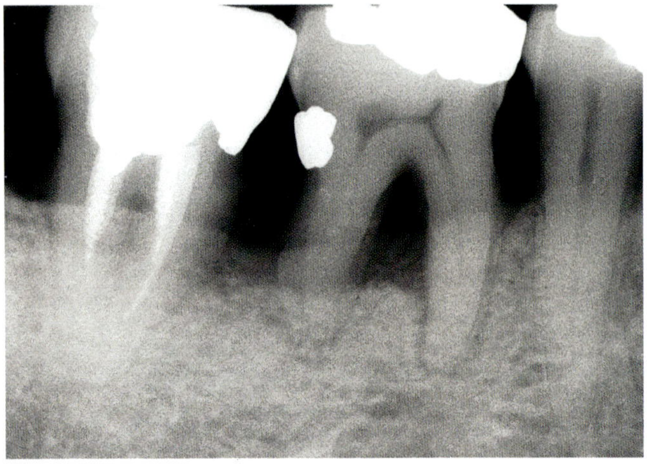

Fig 6-8c Eleven years later, destruction in the furcation has worsened. The mesial septum is unchanged.

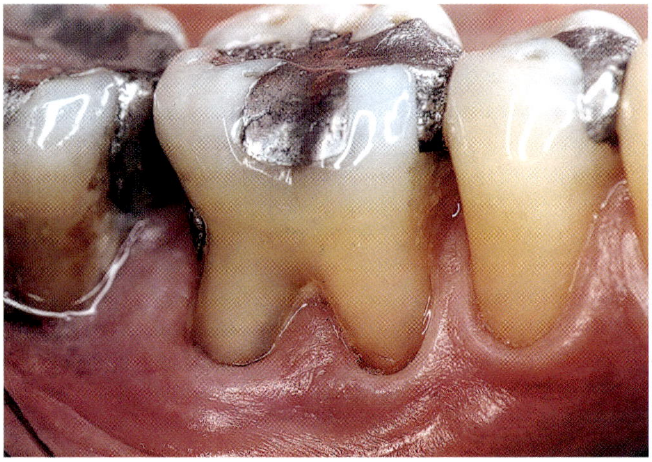

Fig 6-8d The tooth is functional, and despite difficult plaque control, gingival inflammation remains limited.

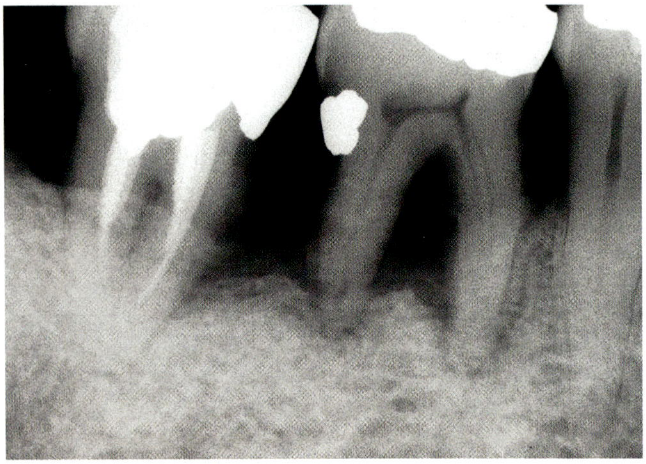

Fig 6-8e Fourteen years after periodontal treatment, controlling inflammation has become very difficult. Both molars are extracted.

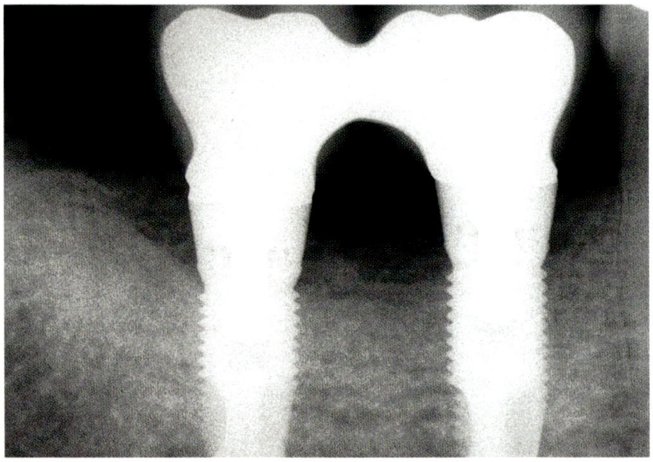

Fig 6-8f Implant rehabilitation is completed. Note bone tissue around implants and premolar. This conservative approach allowed for both teeth to remain in place for 14 years without damage to periodontal tissue or neighboring teeth.

Mobile teeth and splinting

Tooth mobility is a good indicator of periodontal function. It can also represent a possible aggravating factor for periodontal disease (Giargia and Lindhe 1997). Mobility is considered pathologic when periodonal ligament anchorage is modified; this occurs in periodontitis where an enlargement of periodontal ligament space occurs. Weakening of periodontal support tissue is caused by inflammatory destruction. Alteration of periodontal ligament tissue is due to inflammatory congestion and leads to slight tooth egression. Both of these mechanisms are involved in tooth mobility. Mobility indicates a transient or permanent change in periodontal physiology. Mobility and migration are signs of periodontitis that vary with the degree of severity.

Improvement or a complete reversal of mobility and migration may occur after treatment is concluded. On the other hand, when response to treatment is deemed insufficient, it may be necessary to resort to adjunctive therapeutic modalities, such as splinting (Fig 6-9), orthodontic treatment (see Fig 6-4), or extraction (Fig 6-10). Persistence of mobile teeth that interfere with function or plaque control represents a local aggravating factor.

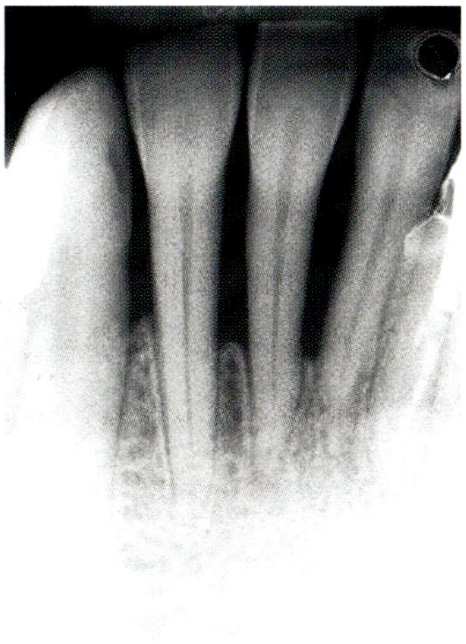

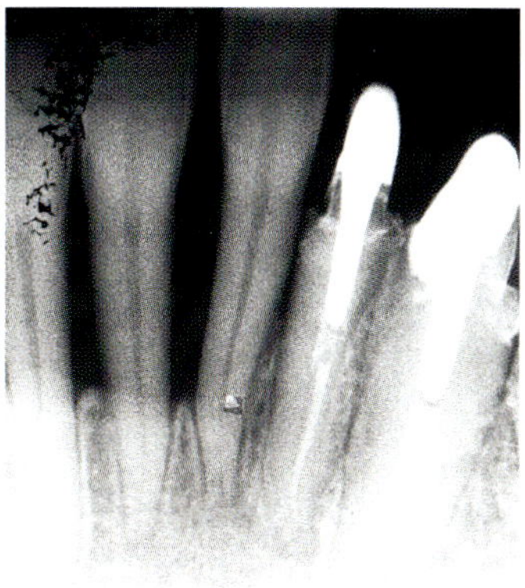

Figs 6-9a and 6-9b Incisor mobility interferes with function and renders plaque control difficult. This is a good indication for splinting.

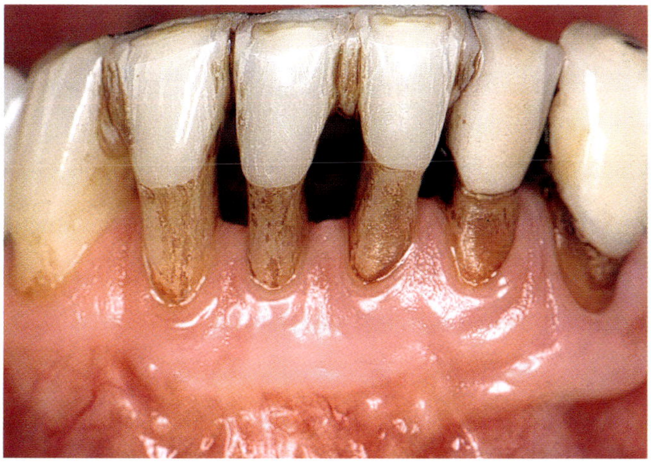

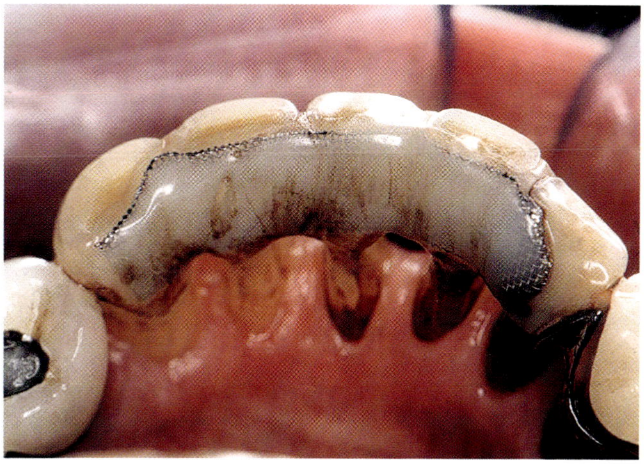

Figs 6-9c and 6-9d The splint consisted of an Ellmann device bonded with composite and was placed in 1981; it remained in place 20 years later.

Mobile teeth and implants

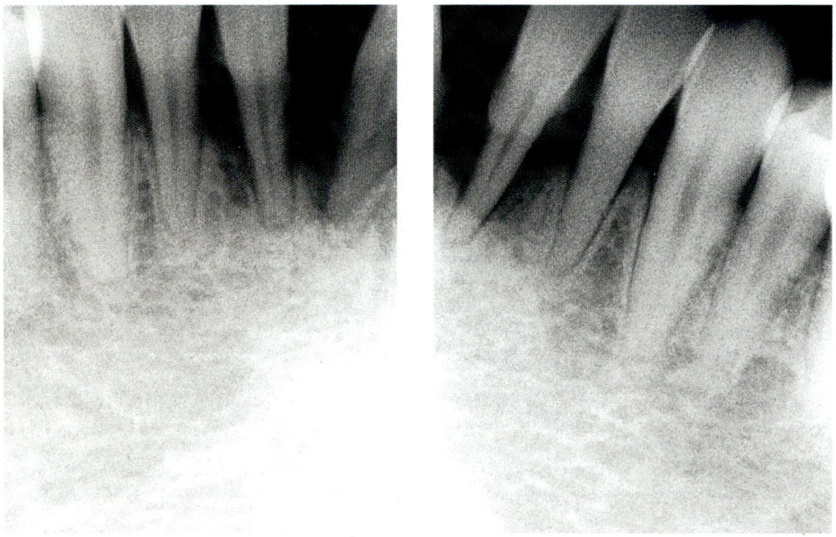

Figs 6-10a and 6-10b Terminal periodontitis is localized at the mandibular incisors. Both central incisors are no longer functional.

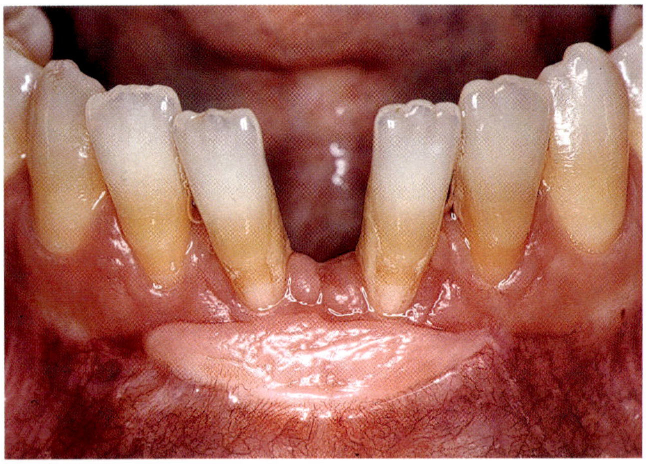

Figs 6-10c Primary interincisal diastema. An implant-based solution is preferred to the use of a splinting device with abutments on both canines.

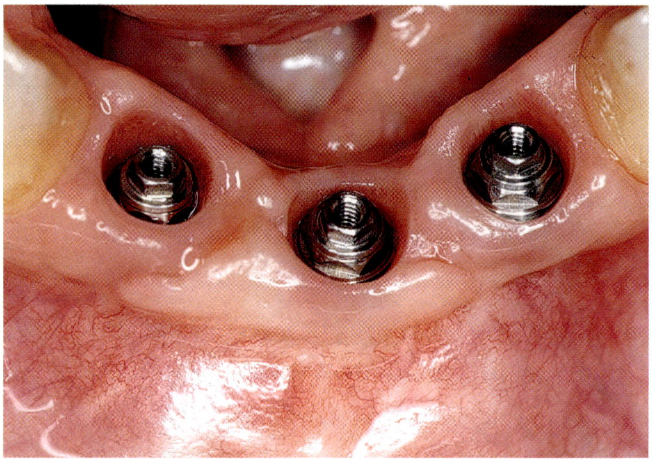

Fig 6-10d Three implants in place.

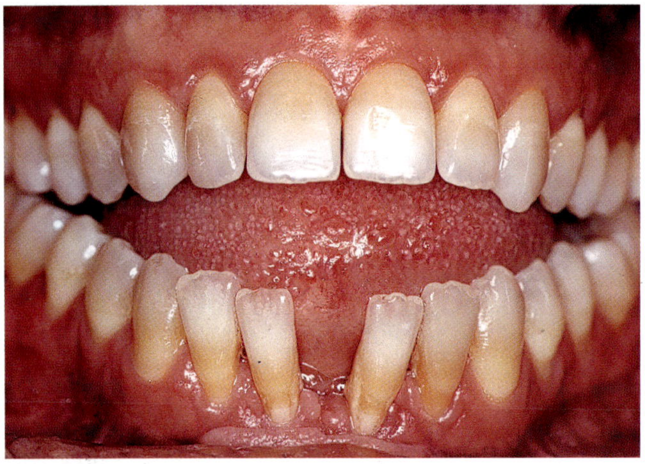

Fig 6-10e Initial clinical situation. Note the macroglossic tongue associated with anterior open bite.

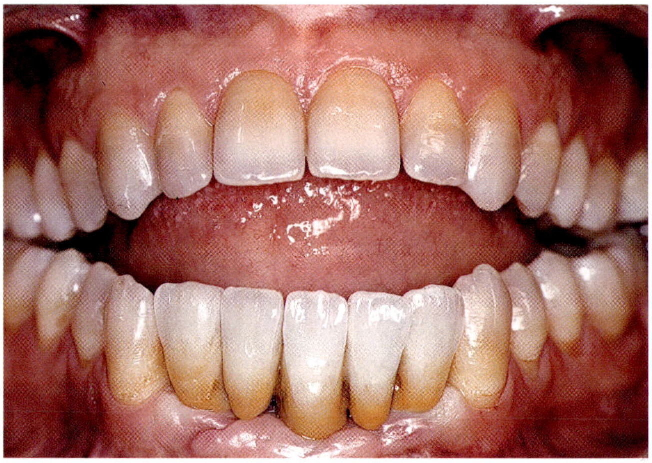

Fig 6-10f Implant-prosthetic rehabilitation with five mandibular incisors.

High-Risk Patients

Genetic predisposition factors

Today, it is clear that for most patients suffering from periodontal disease, consistent plaque control by mechanical elimination of bacterial deposits is sufficient to maintain periodontal health. However, there are certain patients who seem to present other risk factors. Some of these cannot be altered; this is the case with genetic factors. Others are simply difficult to eliminate and may include acquired factors, such as tobacco use and stress, or systemic disease, such as diabetes. All of these factors increase host vulnerability to infection. High-risk patients represent 7% to 15% of the general population; these patients develop severe cases of destructive periodontitis (Johnson et al 1988).

The periodontitis susceptibility test (PST) screens for a specific interleukin-1genotype that has been associated with increased secretion rates of interleukin-1b. This protein stimulates the production of a variety of collagenases involved in tissue destruction (Caffesse et al 2000). Interleukin-1b is thought to play a role in the early onset of inflammatory signs or in disease severity, in combination with other factors. In PST-positive individuals, there is an increased risk for developing periodontal disease between ages 30 and 60 (Kornman et al 1997). Patients from this group feature microbiota with higher levels of pathogenicity than PST-negative control subjects, and they present higher destruction rates (Socransky et al 2000). Also, patients from this group are 2.7 times more likely to lose their teeth during periodontal maintenance. Smoking has also been shown to be a significant risk factor, since it increases the likelihood for losing teeth during supportive therapy by a factor of 2.7 (McGuire and Nunn 1999).

PST-positive status and use of tobacco products can account for 80% of periodontal disease variability.

Treatment response for patients testing positive for the PST test is the same as that for patients with a negative PST result: Regeneration rates at 1 year after surgery is the same for both patient categories. In contrast, follow-up studies of these same patients performed 1 to 4 years after surgery shows twice as much attachment loss in the PST-positive group than in the PST-negative group (de Sanctis and Zuchelli 2000).

Subjects who test positive for the PST are likely to present earlier onset of periodontal disease and are generally more periodontally fragile than subjects who tested negative. They respond to treatment in a similar fashion, but there is a higher risk for disease recurrence. Therefore, they should be followed more closely during maintenance therapy.

Clinical use of the PST

Patient presenting with advanced chronic periodontitis or aggressive periodontitis

A positive result of the PST confirms a predisposition to periodontal disease. Treatment should be more aggressive both in terms of plaque control and in the choice of techniques directed at correcting difficult sites, for example, surgical elimination of deep pockets. Teeth with the lowest periodontal risk are preferable as prosthetic abutments. When dealing with deep sites that bleed on probing, such as deep osseous or furcation lesions, or mobile teeth, implant solutions are often the best long-term option. Once periodontal disease is globally controlled, the infectious risk is low. Periodontal maintenance should be intensified.

Patients with a family history of periodontal disease

Screening for periodontal susceptibility in young adults may help inform subjects who are at higher risk for developing periodontal disease. This is a significant means for motivating these patients toward treatment. These patients require specific, customized treatment strategies designed to prevent the onset of periodontal disease. Associated risk factors should also be considered.

PST sampling

To collect a sample for the PST, a sterile brush is rubbed for 20 to 30 seconds in a regular circular motion against the buccal mucous membrane. After the brush is air dried for 1 minute, it is placed in a test tube before being sent off to the lab. Analysis is performed on DNA strands. No special measures need to be taken for expected delays.

Smoking and periodontitis

Tobacco smoking is an important risk factor in the initiation and progression of periodontal disease. Smoking is a negative factor for treatment outcome. Many studies have found evidence of immunologic and cell dysfunction associated with tobacco use. In smokers, immune response, phagocytosis, chemotaxis of polymorphonuclear leukocytes, vascular regeneration, and healing mechanisms all seem to be altered.

In heavy smokers (subjects who smoke more than 20 cigarettes a day), attachment and bone losses are more than twice those found in occasional smokers (Grossi et al 1994; Grossi et al 1995). Heavy smokers are found to have more attachment loss, more missing teeth, and deeper probing depths. Interestingly, they have fewer sites that bleed on probing compared to nonsmokers or ex-smokers. Attachment losses on palatal surfaces of maxillary teeth or on mandibular anterior teeth are generally more severe. This seems to be the consequence of cigarette-induced local effects (Haffajee and Socransky 2001). Older individuals who are smokers tend to lose more teeth than do nonsmokers (Axelsson et al 1998). In vitro there is evidence of synergistic actions between tobacco-derived cotinine and toxins derived from periodontopathic species such as *P intermedia*, *Prevotella nigriscens*, or *P gingivalis* (Sayers et al 1999). This may explain why tobacco increases the severity of periodontal disease.

Scabbia et al (2001) investigated the negative effect of tobacco on tissue healing. These authors stated that the pocket depth reductions and attachment gains observed among nonsmokers after periodontal flap surgery did not occur in smokers. The potential for a reparative response is significantly reduced in smokers.

Treatment of patients who smoke is often a cause for disappointment. These subjects should be strongly encouraged to quit. The fact that ex-smokers have better treatment outcomes should be used to motivate smokers in their attempt to reduce cigarette smoking or quit altogether.

> Disease severity is increased among smokers; treatment response is reduced; subgingival bacteria, especially gram-negative species, tend to be more numerous; and tissue healing is delayed. Antibiotic therapy is often indicated and proves efficient. Quitting smoking is an integral part of periodontal treatment.

Diabetes

Diabetic patients are two or three times more likely to develop periodontal disease than are nondiabetic subjects. However, flora composition is identical in diabetics and nondiabetics.

When diabetes is controlled, patients respond well to treatment and the risk for developing periodontitis is the same as in nondiabetic subjects. In patients with uncontrolled diabetes, however, severity of periodontal disease increases and tissue destruction is more extensive. Diabetic patients presenting with periodontal disease should be systematically treated; those who present aggressive or refractory forms of periodontal disease should be referred for proper assessment of diabetic status.

Stress

Stress has behavioral consequences and thereby may induce important negative changes in habit patterns. A stressed smoker will tend to smoke more and a stressed clencher will clench more. Likewise, plaque control and oral hygiene are reduced.

Prognosis and Long-term Outcome

7

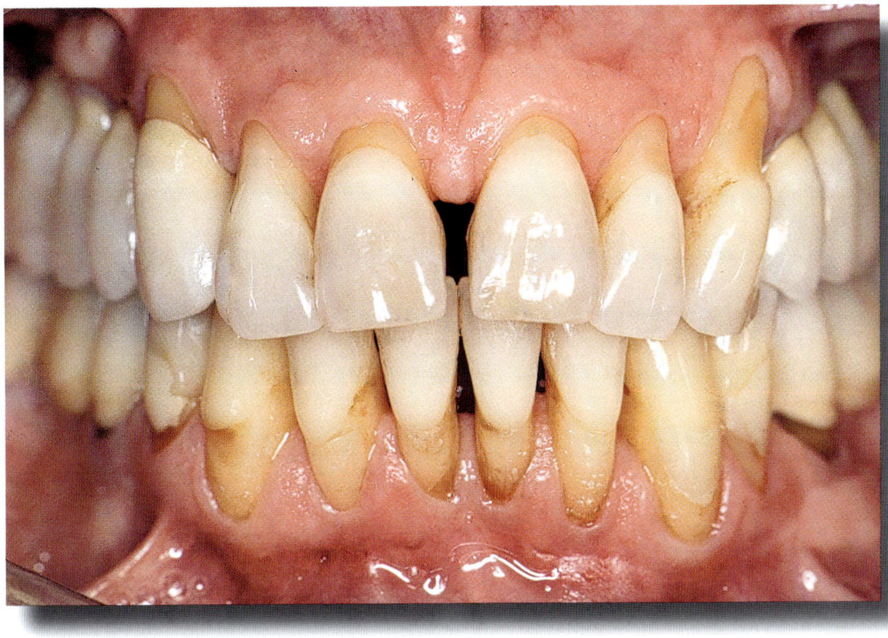

Limits to Conservative Treatment

When managing treatment of advanced periodontal disease, successful conditions are fulfilled when periodontal tissue is stabilized throughout the whole dentition. Managing periodontal disease means:

- Successful treatment of infection
- Effective restoration of function and esthetics
- Prevention of recurrence
- Effective recurrence management when necessary
- Carrying out the best suited maintenance therapy program

To reach these goals, the available tools are:

- Increasingly precise diagnostic tests
- More targeted treatment protocols
- More efficient regeneration techniques
- Better assessment methods
- Less traumatic prosthetic treatments

In the context of these developments, what goals for periodontal management are realistic? When dealing with advanced periodontitis, teeth presenting significant periodontal tissue destruction should be preserved during the preliminary treatment phase. This approach proceeds from a principle based on an optimistic outcome that can be applied in cases of aggressive periodontitis as well as advanced chronic periodontitis, on the condition that severity factors can actually be modified. A definitive prognosis for these teeth should be made during or at the end of treatment. Maintain or extract? Each tooth should be evaluated continuously throughout the course of treatment (and afterward) while specific treatment modalities are being applied. When successful conditions have been achieved as previously defined, the choice of tooth conservation is validated.

In assessing risk factors linked to tooth conservation, three points should be considered:

- Tooth conservation should not, in any way, compromise the prognosis of other teeth.
- Tooth conservation should not involve a more unfavorable prognosis than any other treatment option.
- Tooth conservation should be the best treatment option for the patient in the long run.

Advanced, Locally Terminal Periodontitis

The patient in Fig 7-1 presented no occlusal contacts on the left side. Masticatory function was difficult and occurred only on the right side. The maxillary right second premolar and first molar were tender to percussion and presented Class III mobility. Anterior function was disturbed as well, with significant incisor mobility and displacements. There was a significant esthetic handicap and a disturbed smile. Local factors predominated and were dental, periodontal, anatomic, functional, and esthetic in nature. The preferred treatment strategy was to preserve all teeth during the course of global periodontal treatment, which proved to be very complex. Periodontal, orthodontic, and orthognathic surgical methods were used in treating this patient.

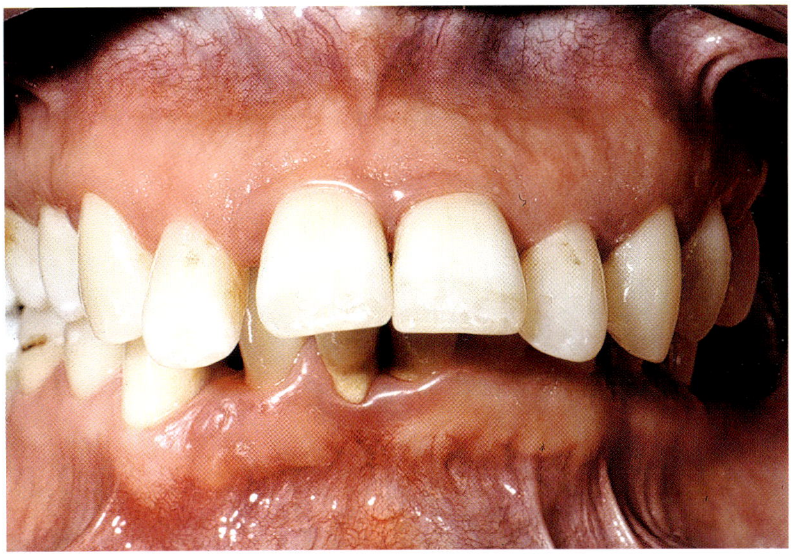

Fig 7-1a Aggressive periodontitis associated with multiple factors in a 40-year-old female patient.

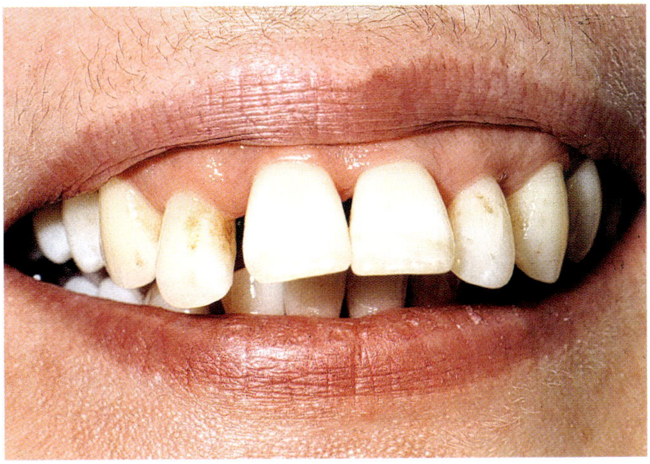

Fig 7-1b Absence of occlusal contacts on the left, tooth mobility, and incisor migration are apparent. The smile is affected.

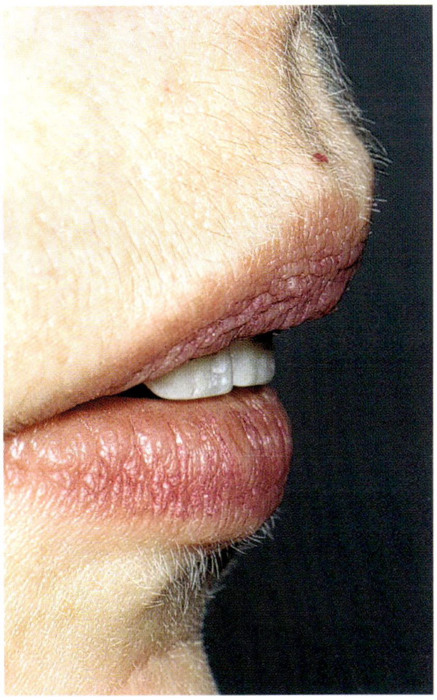

Fig 7-1c Lip closure is difficult.

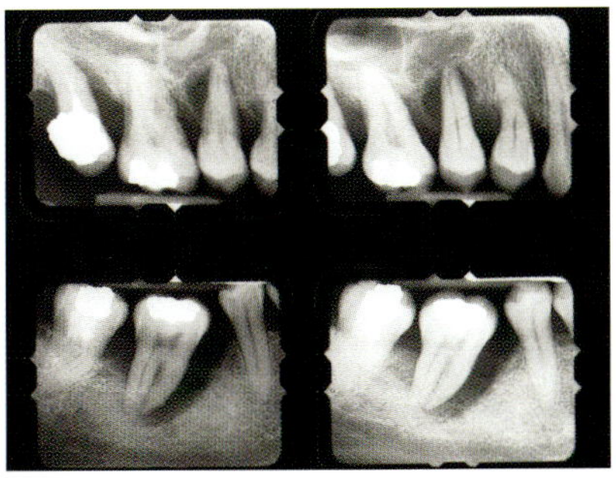

Fig 7-1d The mandibular right second molar is inclined mesially and the maxillary right second premolar presents Class II mobility. Both teeth present terminal bone destruction.

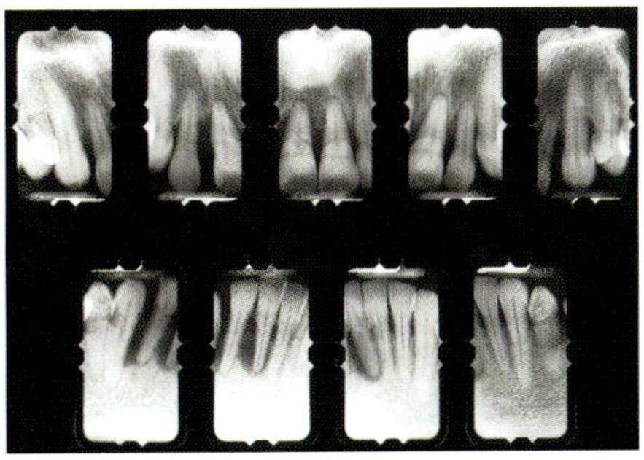

Fig 7-1e Locally, attachment losses and periodontal destruction are extremely significant.

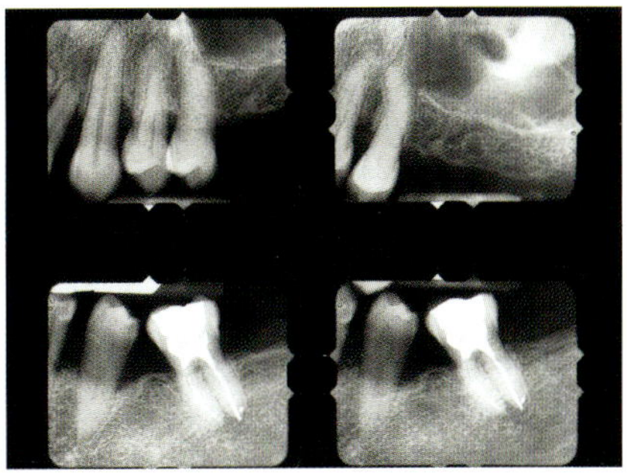

Fig 7-1f The maxillary left molars and the mandibular left first molar no longer exist. The mandibular second molar is inclined mesially.

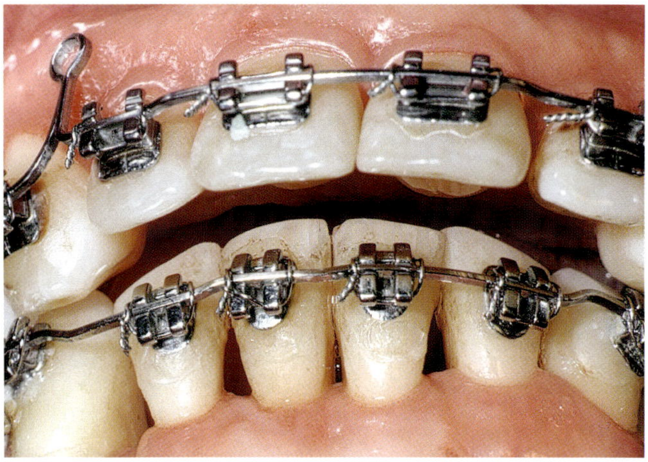

Fig 7-1g Periodontal treatment, consisting of mechanical, antibiotic, and surgical treatment involving a local grafting procedure, is finalized. Orthodontic treatment is performed to correct dental displacements. Note the anteroposterior shift between both arches.

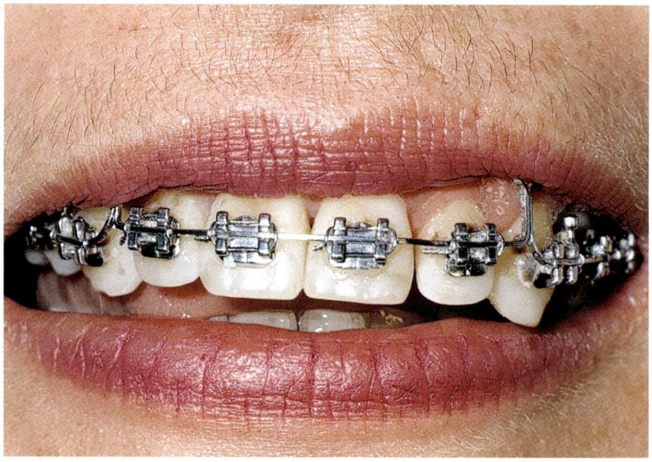

Fig 7-1h The maxillary occlusal plane is oblique on the left side. Also on the left side, there are no dental contacts.

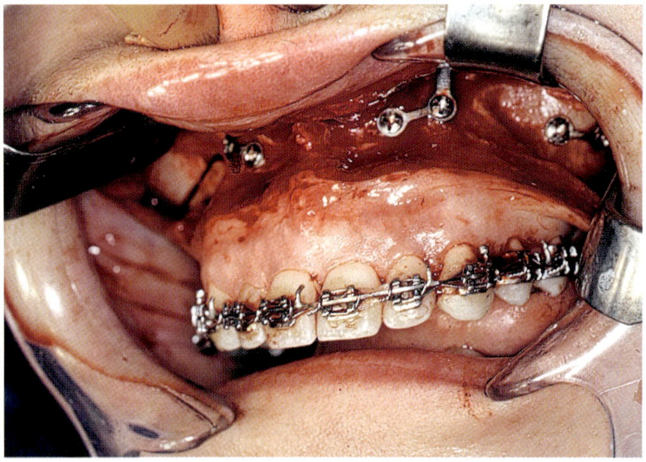

Fig 7-1i Orthognathic surgery rotates the maxilla to reestablish a horizontal occlusal plane.

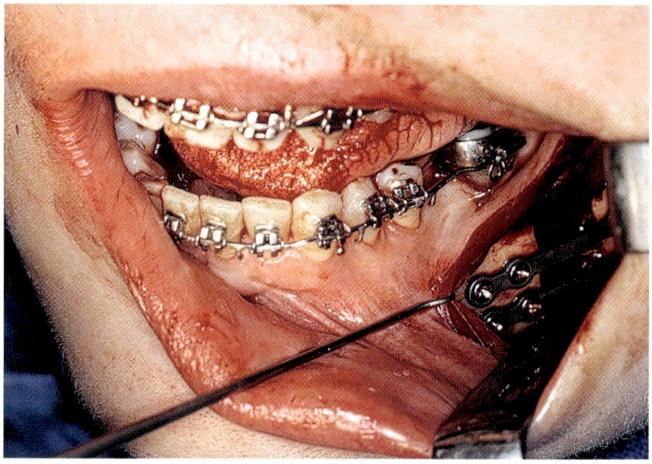

Fig 7-1j The discrepancy is further reduced by mandibular advancement, which reestablishes anterior and left-side contacts between both arches, all of which were absent prior to the procedure.

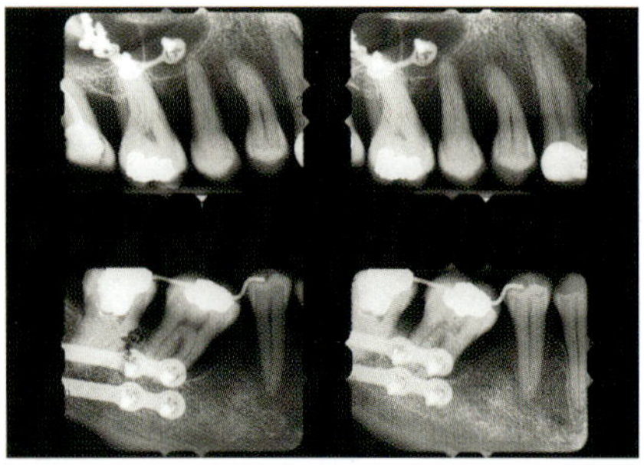

Fig 7-1k Five years after the start of treatment, the maxillary right second premolar and the mandibular right second molar are in place and remain functional. Fixed prosthetic rehabilitation will be considered later.

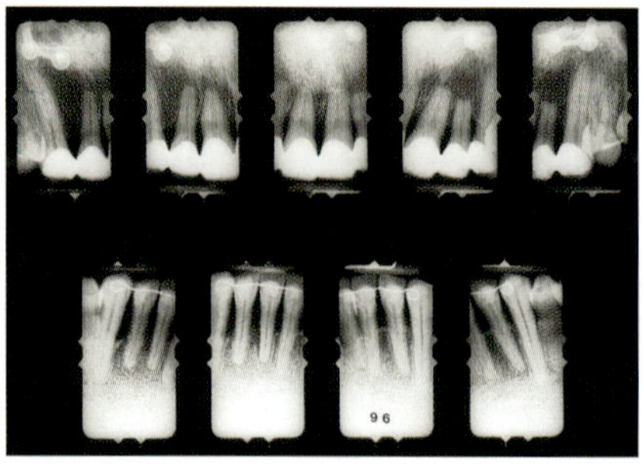

Fig 7-1l Slight root resorption is seen after orthodontic treatment. Note the favorable response in all areas of the periodontium, as well as the repair processes that have occurred around the incisors.

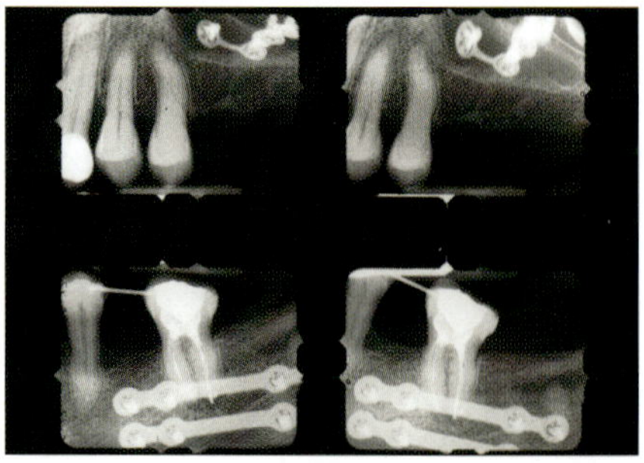

Fig 7-1m The mandibular left second molar is orthodontically shifted before being integrated as an abutment in a prosthetic reconstruction.

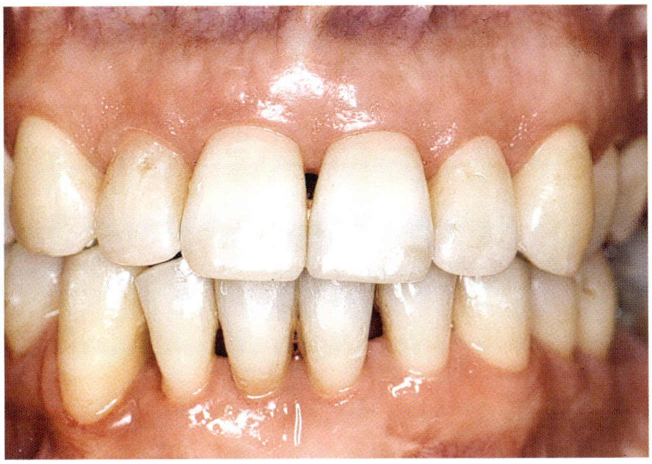

Fig 7-1n End of active therapy. The tissues display signs of periodontal health. In the mandibular incisor region, gingival reinforcement was achieved by performing an epithelial-connective tissue graft.

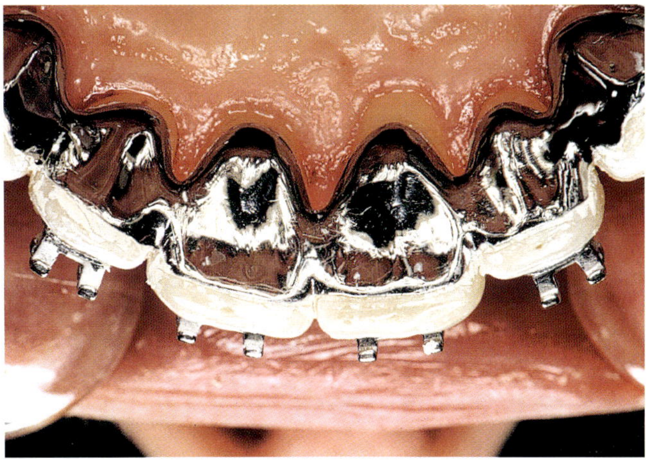

Fig 7-1o Bonded splinting device from canine to canine.

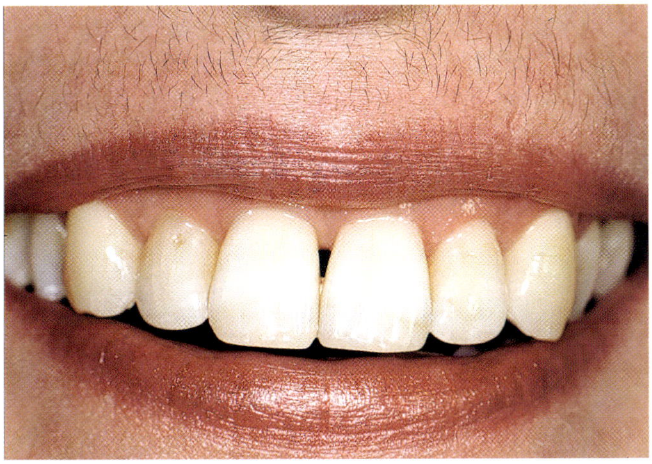

Fig 7-1p The patient's smile has been recovered.

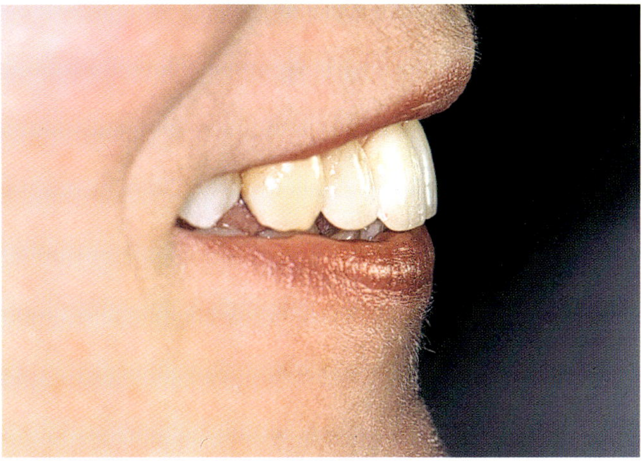

Fig 7-1q Esthetic outcome is very satisfactory.

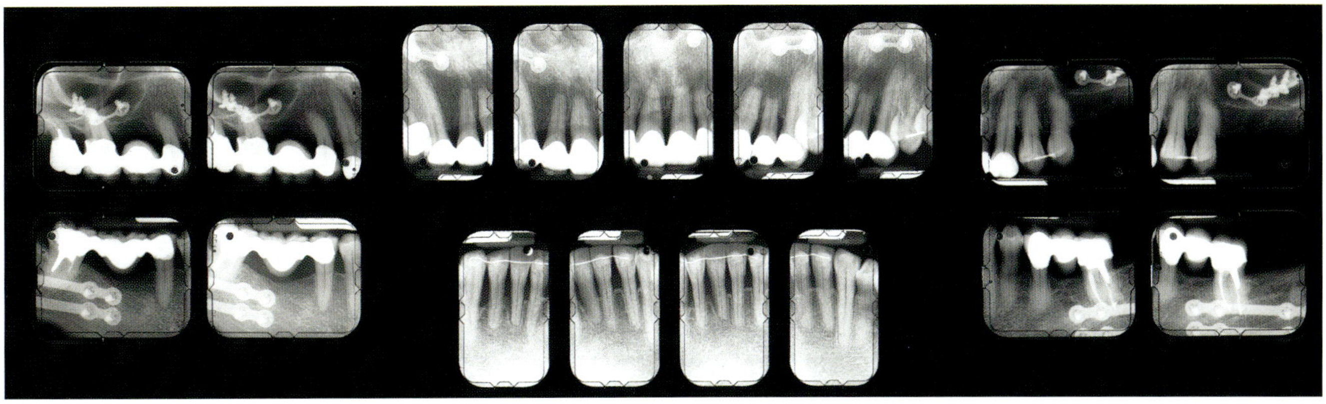

Figs 7-1r to 7-1t Radiographic evaluation 10 years after the start of treatment confirms periodontal health. Fixed prosthetic restorations have been placed in the posterior regions. Two implants are scheduled to be placed in the maxillary left posterior quadrant.

At about the same time as the radiographic evaluation, the patient was subjected to a periodontitis susceptibility test, which was negative. According to this test, the patient is not at high risk for developing periodontal disease. Severity factors are bacterial or local; response to treatment is very favorable, and periodontal maintenance is scheduled to be performed on a regular basis.

Implants and Risk of Infection

Peri-implant flora

In completely edentulous patients, pathogenic bacterial species are undetectable. After implants are placed, pathogenic microbiota remain absent. When samples are collected around implants, microbial populations are shown to consist essentially in gram-positive, beneficial, nonpathogenic bacteria. On the other hand, in partially edentulous patients, flora collected from implant sites is similar to that found around natural teeth. Natural teeth may act as reservoir sites and lead to secondary colonization of dental implant sites by pathogenic species (Quirynen and Listgarten 1990). Thus, periodontal pockets from residual teeth become potential infectious foci for dental implants (Fig 7-2). Accordingly, the same pathogenic bacterial species have been observed in infectious peri-implant tissues (Mombelli and Lang 1994).

Consequences of plaque accumulation around implants

Peri-implant mucositis is a reversible, inflammatory reaction to increased amounts of plaque and is limited to the soft tissues adjacent to the functional implant. This phenomenon is frequent, though it seldom evolves into peri-implantitis.

Peri-implantitis is an inflammatory reaction of infectious origin that occurs in the soft tissue adjacent to the implant, with subsequent loss of bone tissue around the implant. This leads to chronicity and episodic inflammatory reactivation. Left untreated, this inflammatory reaction threatens implant osseointegration and may lead to loss of the implant. Such treatment failures have not been reported in edentulous patients. However, the opportunities for implant placement in deep sites or in partially edentulous situations are more common than in the past. This warrants caution in posing the indications for implant placement, even though the proportion of implants lost to peri-implantitis is low compared to the proportion of those lost for biomechanical reasons.

Periodontal infection and peri-implantitis

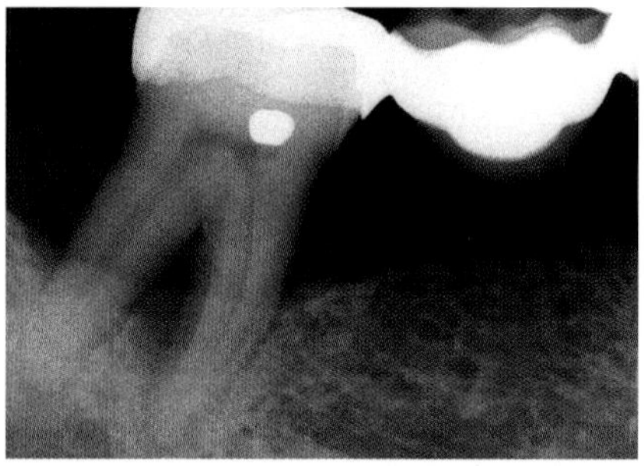

Fig 7-2a Nonstabilized periodontitis in a 64-year-old female patient who smokes. A deep pocket in a molar furcation is present. There is a history of periodic infectious episodes in this region, where plaque scores are significant.

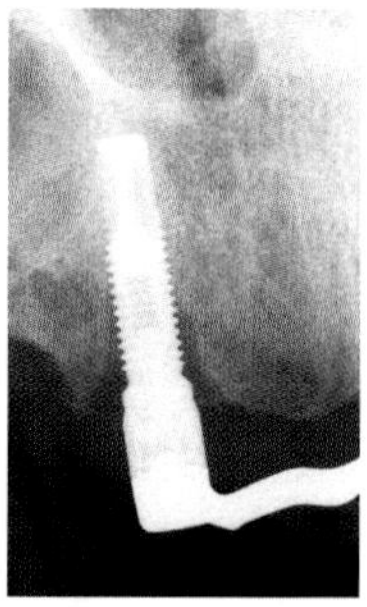

Fig 7-2b Peri-implantitis associated with the presence of *Porphyromonas gingivalis* (55%) and *Tannerella forsythensis* (7%) and concomitant commensal infection (high plaque scores plus *Prevotella intermedia, Peptostreptococcus micros,* and *Fusobacterium nucleatum*). Bone destruction is significant, and the implant is mobile. It was subsequently removed.

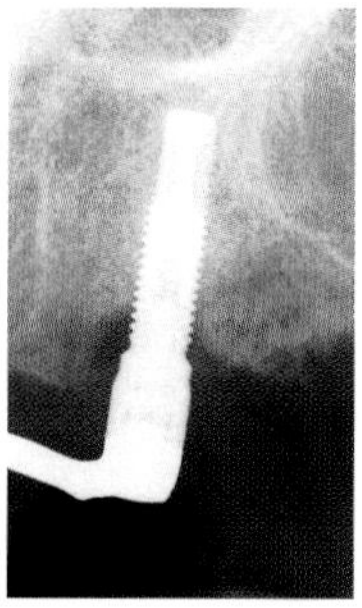

Fig 7-2c This second implant also presents signs of peri-implantitis, but bone destruction is less severe and the implant is less mobile. Conservation of the implant is attempted. A periodontal infectious source is probably responsible for peri-implant infection.

When should the decision to extract be made? In cases of severe periodontal disease, indications for extraction are frequent (Table 7-1). Extraction may be necessary for teeth that continue to undergo attachment loss despite periodontal treatment, or for teeth affected by generalized terminal periodontitis (Fig 7-3).

Table 7-1 Suggestions for periodontal preparation prior to implant surgery

Diagnosis	Course of treatment	Infectious risk	Periodontal preparation
Generalized terminal periodontitis	1. Full-mouth extractions and placement of removable complete denture. 2. Implant surgery.	No pathogenic bacteria. No infectious risk.	No periodontal preparation is necessary before implant surgery.
Advanced, locally terminal periodontitis	1. Single- or multiple-tooth extractions at beginning of periodontal treatment. 2. Implant surgery.	Risk is high if implant surgery is initiated too early in treatment; risk is low if surgery is performed after periodontal preparation.	Etiologic periodontal treatment, microbiologic screening, and antibiotic treatment. Implant surgery (embedded implants) may be performed before periodontal surgery.
Generalized terminal periodontitis (see Fig 7-3)	1. Multiple teeth are compromised. Some are temporarily preserved as prosthetic abutments for transitional prosthesis. 2. Implantation is done in two steps.	Saved teeth are potential infectious foci. Risk is high if implant surgery is performed before periodontal surgery.	Etiologic periodontal treatment, microbiologic screening, antibiotic treatment, and periodontal surgery for teeth temporarily used as abutments.

Deep periodontal pockets represent potential infectious foci. As a general rule, implant surgery should not be carried out in the presence of such pockets.

Terminal periodontitis and implants

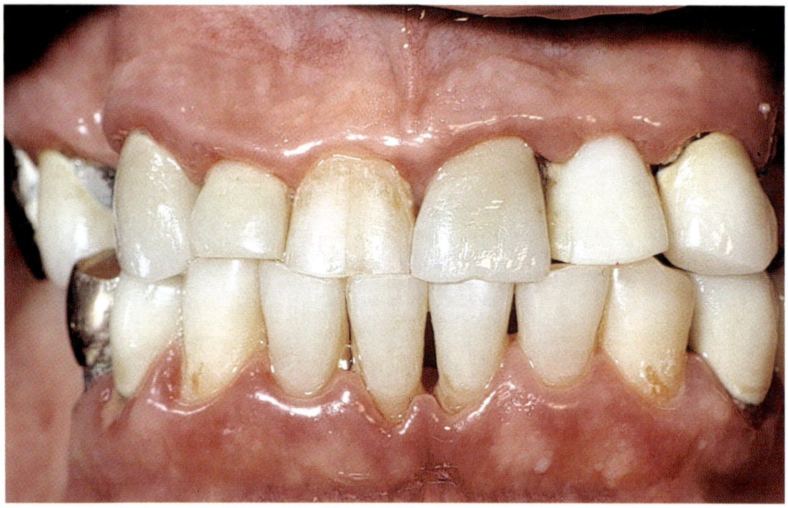

Fig 7-3a Advanced chronic periodontitis in a 53-year-old, otherwise healthy, nonsmoking male patient. Pathogenic species, including *P gingivalis* (8%), are present. Multiple severity factors are determined.

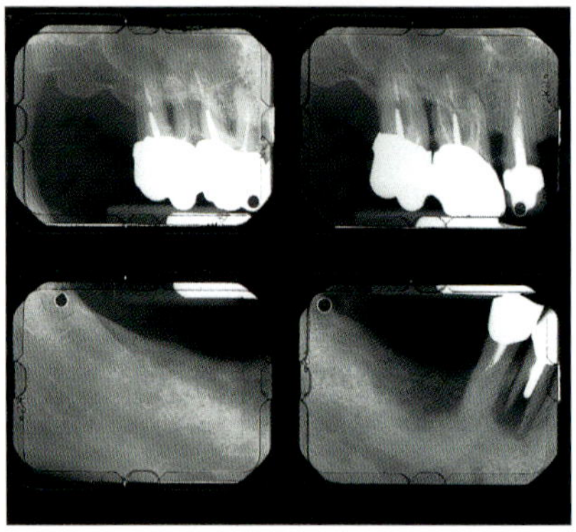

Fig 7-3b In remaining molars, destruction involves furcation regions (Class III). Mobility is significant, and the mandibular right first premolar is fractured.

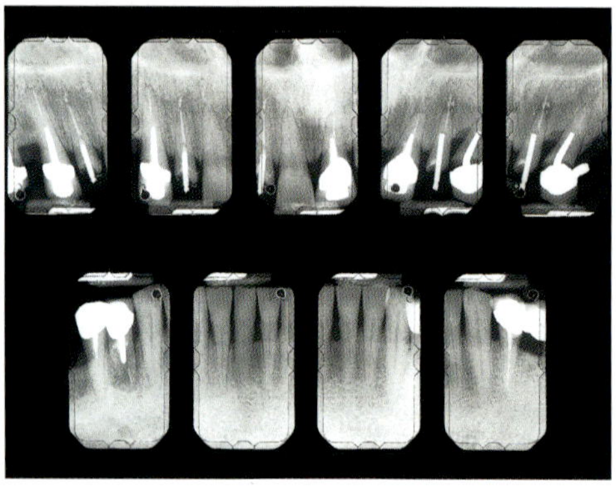

Fig 7-3c Numerous local factors (dental, functional, and iatrogenic) account for the extent of destruction. The maxillary left canine is fractured.

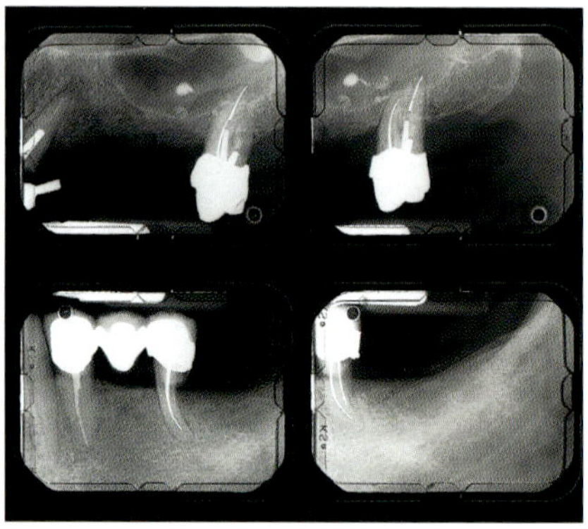

Fig 7-3d Similar destruction is noted around the maxillary left second molar.

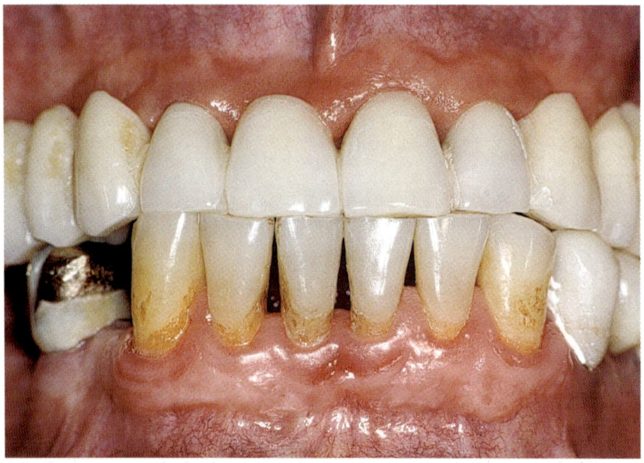

Fig 7-3e The treatment strategy consisted of periodontal therapy and fixed prosthetic and implant rehabilitation over the entire maxilla and bilateral mandibular posterior sextants. After the first phase of periodontal therapy, a fixed partial denture was fabricated with the Yuodelis technique (Yuodelis 1980). This allowed for the redefinition of functional occlusal guidance schemes.

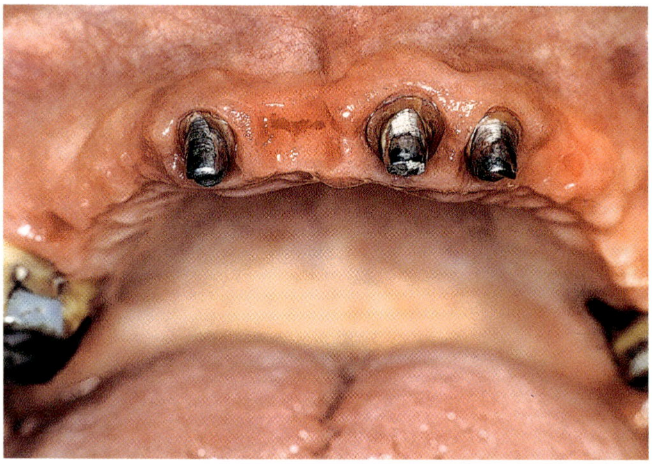

Fig 7-3f Periodontal therapy allows for provisional use of favorably distributed abutments where periodontal tissue is severely compromised (maxillary right first and second molars, both lateral incisors, and the left central incisor and second molar). Periodontal treatment consists of local treatment, antibiotic therapy (amoxicillin), and periodontal surgery.

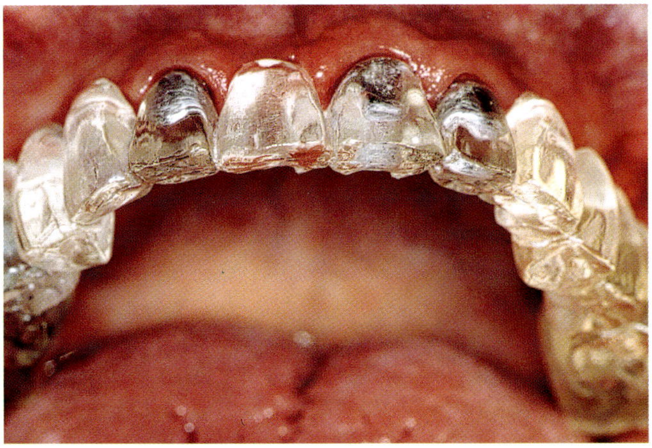

Fig 7-3g A surgical template is fabricated according to the multiunit provisional restoration. During the first phase of implant surgery, five implants are placed.

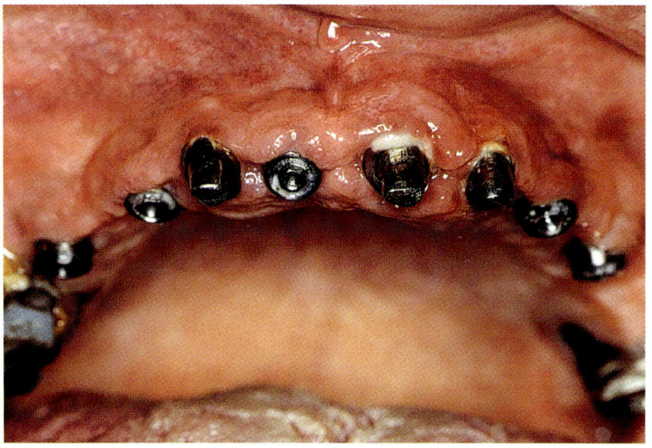

Fig 7-3h At stage 2 the healing screw is placed; definitive abutments are placed a few weeks later. Impressions can then be made.

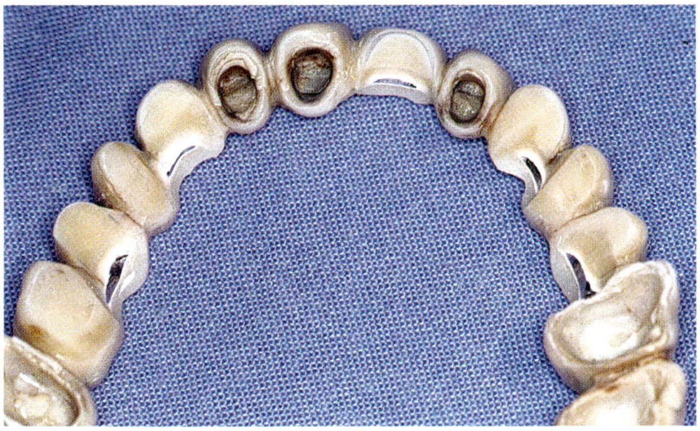

Fig 7-3i At each step the provisional multiunit restoration can be readapted as necessary.

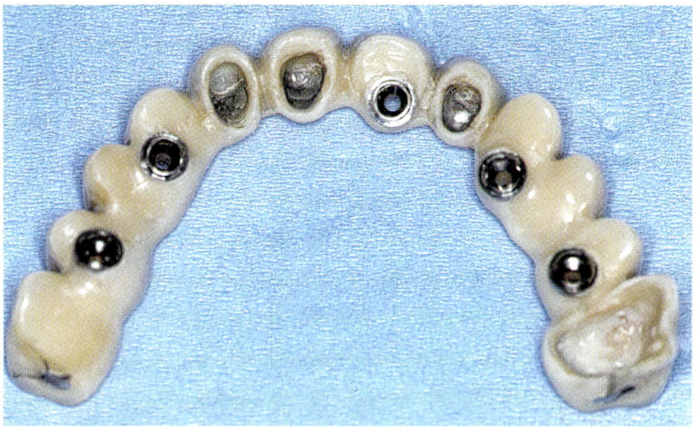

Fig 7-3j On the working model, the provisional multiunit restoration, initially used for mounting on the articulator, is transferred onto the implants. The abutment teeth are extracted, and new implants are placed in the position of the left central incisor and in both tuberosities.

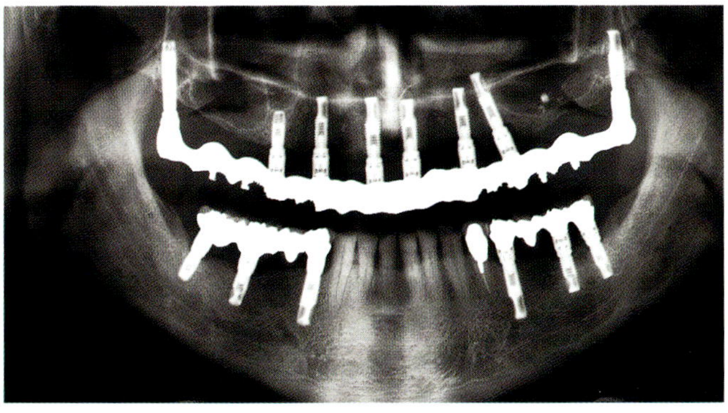

Fig 7-3k Prosthetic rehabilitation in place. The tuberosity implants act as posterior abutments, thus avoiding distal prosthetic extensions.

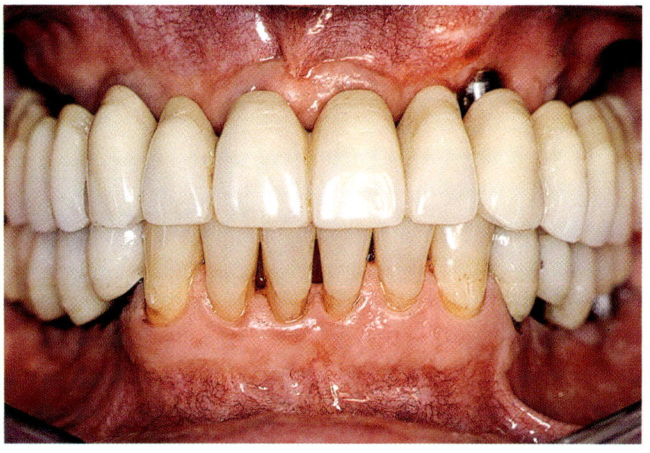

Fig 7-3l Clinical situation 5 years after the end of treatment. Global treatment stretched over a period of 2 years. Provisionalization with fixed prosthetic constructions was continuous during treatment, including the periods of implant surgery. This represents exceptional comfort both for the patient and for the practitioner.

Success in such treatments is only possible if periodontal disease is monitored and if compromised teeth, which may be preserved for several months, do not present infectious foci from which pathogenic bacteria may disseminate to nearby implant sites.

Periodontal Maintenance

Periodontal treatment involves controlling the different parameters of disease, reestablishing a balance between bacterial microbiota and periodontal tissue, and finally, restoring attachment tissue stability in all areas of the dentition. The main objective of supportive therapy is to prevent recurrence of disease. This occurs when, in any given site, attachment loss recurs as a consequence of local modifications and/or a change in the patient's ability to control the accumulation of plaque. There is no single criterion on which to base the strategy used to prevent recurrence. The prime objective is to support periodontal health.

Repeated gingival bleeding is a significant indicator of periodontal disease recurrence (Lang et al 1986). Sites with higher probing depths after treatment are at greater risk for aggravation than sites with lower probing scores (Listgarten et al 1991).

Maintenance therapy is started after completion of active periodontal therapy. Maintenance therapy should be continued on a lifelong basis, at intervals deemed appropriate for each individual patient, and should be performed around all teeth and implants. Periodontal maintenance is an extension of active periodontal therapy (American Academy of Periodontology 2000).

Methods

Procedures involved in periodontal maintenance include collecting or carrying out:

- Past medical history and history of periodontal disease
- Radiographic evaluation
- Soft tissue examination
- Dental examination
- Periodontal examination
- Review and assessment of patient's plaque control
- Removal of microbial flora from sulcular or pocket areas
- Scaling and planing where indicated
- Tooth polishing

These methods are used at regular intervals to assist the patient in maintaining periodontal health. During maintenance therapy, periodontal disease can be monitored because etiologic factors have previously been reduced or eliminated. Maintenance represents a distinct, additional phase of treatment and follows active treatment stage. When recurrence is suspected, active care may be resumed.

Therapeutic goals

The objective of periodontal maintenance is twofold:

- To prevent recurrence and progression of periodontal disease in patients who have previously been treated for gingivitis or periodontitis
- To reduce the incidence of tooth loss while simultaneously restoring a functional dentition and replacing missing teeth

Treatment considerations

- *Clinical examination*: To be compared with baseline findings.
- *Radiographic examination*.

- *Reevaluation*: Entails clinical and radiographic evaluation of disease, as well as assessment of plaque control effectiveness.
- *Communication*: Involves informing the patient of the various observed changes. This aspect of reevaluation also may involve consulting with other health care providers who may be asked to provide additional therapy or participate in the periodontal maintenance program.
- *Therapy*: Includes removal of supragingival and subgingival plaque and calculus, antibiotic therapy as indicated, and surgical treatment in recurrent sites. When reintervention is necessary, the clinician should consider resuming oral hygiene recommendations, controlling risk factors, such as tobacco use, and increasing the frequency of maintenance therapy.
- *Periodontal maintenance schedule:* For most patients with periodontal disease, follow-up visits with scaling and root planing at 3-month intervals have been found to be effective in maintaining gingival health. Depending on the outcome of clinical reevaluation, the frequency of periodontal maintenance visits may be modified, or the patient may be returned to active treatment.
- *Outcomes assessment*: The main objective is long-term maintenance of periodontal health status attained as a result of active therapy. Insufficient periodontal maintenance or noncompliance may result in recurrence or disease progression. Occasionally, despite patient compliance and adequate periodontal maintenance, disease progression may occur. In these cases, additional therapy should be considered.

Individual maintenance therapy

The patient's point of view

"Doctor, thank you, I am very happy with the way my treatment went, even though it took a long time. I have now recovered a feeling of comfort in my teeth, I have no pain, my gums don't bleed anymore, my bad breath problem is gone, and I have no difficulty chewing. Actually, I don't think about my teeth anymore. I guess I am cured." What comes next?

The practitioner's point of view

There is a risk for disease recurrence, and this is all the more likely when treated periodontal disease was severe. The patient should be fully informed: active periodontal maintenance involves both personal and professional care. Maintenance therapy is the only means for efficient monitoring of periodontal disease and should therefore be scrupulously followed. At this point, the patient understands his or her full responsibility in maintaining the periodontal health status established by the practitioner through active treatment.

Daily maintenance therapy

This primarily involves the patient's proficiency in oral hygiene measures. The patient should also be able to detect any signs or episodic manifestations of disease recurrence.

- *Brushing frequency*: Statistically, brushing twice daily and professional follow-up sessions performed every 3 months have been found to effectively stabilize the gingival health of patients with periodontal disease. Patients with advanced forms of periodontitis are more vulnerable: brushing should be performed three times a day. This habit should be acquired during the active phase of treatment and should be continued after active therapy. During active treatment, plaque control effectiveness should be assessed at each visit; this implies that the patient should brush before each visit, and consequently that the patient should brush after each meal. The clinical situation resulting from the cumulative effects of periodontal disease and therapy is favorable to additional plaque accumulation in interdental spaces. This justifies regular brushing after the midday meal.

- *Brushing method and type of toothbrush*: Plaque deposits build up on the surface of gingival tissue, on dental surfaces, and in proximal spaces. The modified Bass method (involving a rolling stroke from the gingiva toward the dental surfaces away from the gingiva) is best suited for access to interproximal regions where plaque control is most difficult. Swift and energetic rinsing should be performed before starting the brushing procedure. A small amount of dentifrice should be placed on a dry toothbrush. Emphasis should be placed on the mechanical action of the brush for cleaning gingival and dental surfaces. The patient should be advised to make 8 to 10 brush movements for efficient removal of dental plaque. All surfaces of all teeth should be brushed. Use of interdental brushes is mandatory for patients with advanced periodontitis, since the risk for recurrence is higher in interproximal areas. After the midday meal, a quick brushing procedure without dentifrice, between two mouth rinses, is generally sufficient to eliminate most plaque deposits. Use of a powered toothbrush allows for better elimination of plaque on mandibular lingual surfaces. On other areas, efficiency of powered toothbrushes is similar to that of manual toothbrushes (Haffajee et al 2001).
- *The interproximal space*: Recurrence most frequently occurs in interproximal spaces. This warrants the use of specific techniques for plaque removal: interdental brushes with adequate dimensions and shapes should be used in these sites. Dental floss may also be used to clean proximal surfaces. The importance of the interdental space needs to be considered at all times, and especially during prosthetic rehabilitation, where biologic width and embrasure form are crucial clinical parameters.
- *Implants and periodontal maintenance*: Bacterial plaque does not adhere as strongly on titanium as it does on mineralized dental surfaces. It is therefore easier to remove plaque from implant surfaces than from dental surfaces. Some prosthetic constructions feature regions where plaque removal is made difficult by complex morphology. Likewise, the subgingival location of some cosmetic elements of these constructions may interfere with adequate plaque control measures.

Special Circumstances

Periodontal disease is usually not painful. The patient should therefore be informed of the nature of the signs or episodic manifestations preceding recurrence of disease progression and attachment loss. The best way for the patient to recognize disease recurrence is to be able to identify and interpret the early symptoms of inflammation:

- Bleeding on probing
- Cold sensitivity
- Heat sensitivity
- Tenderness
- Sensation of having "long teeth"

When any of these symptoms occur, it is important to:

- Check the toothbrush and change if necessary.
- Increase brushing frequency and intensity around the affected site. The patient may apply a chlorhexidine-based mouthwash to the toothbrush. If symptoms do not reverse within a few days, a professional maintenance visit and reevaluation should be scheduled.

Frequency of professional follow-up

The minimum frequency of professional periodontal maintenance is three visits a year. The frequency of these sessions may be increased when indicated. Maintenance planning should be established with the patient's consent, and the patient should fully understand the importance of efficient plaque control.

The Interproximal Space

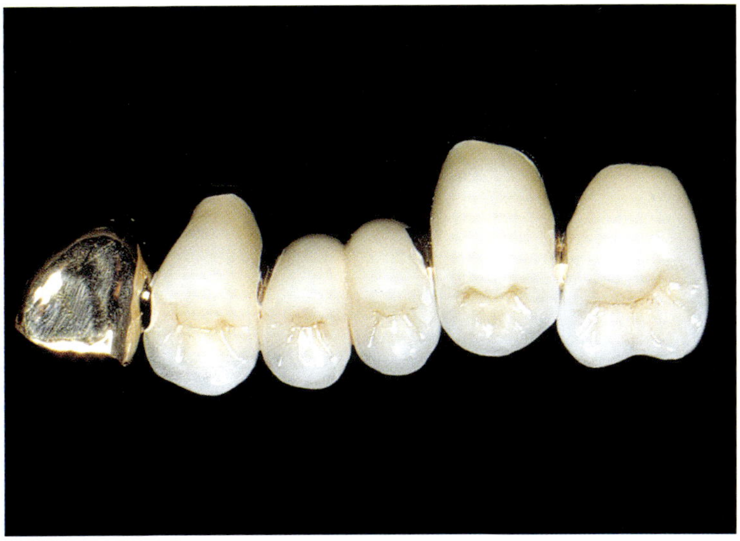

Fig 7-4a This prosthetic restoration respects the biologic space, and its morphologic features are compatible with plaque control measures.

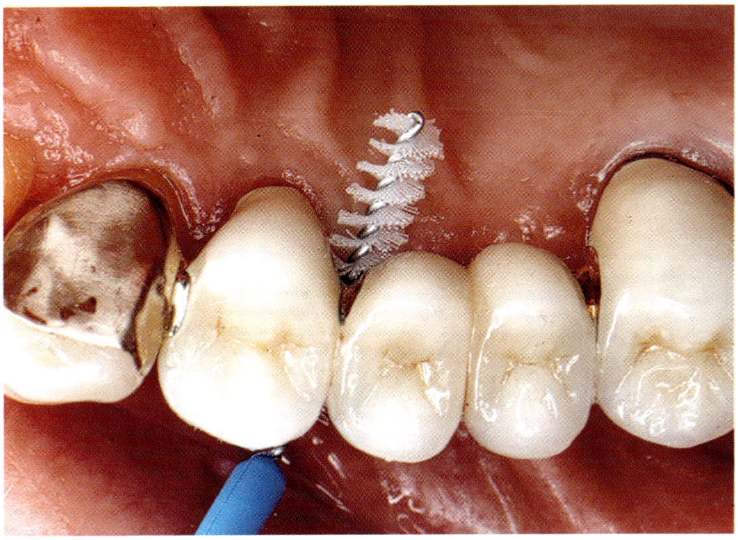

Fig 7-4b Plaque control in the interproximal space requires use of interdental brushes.

Long-term Outcome of Advanced Periodontitis

The combination of strict oral hygiene measures and professional periodontal maintenance therapy has been shown to promote maintenance of periodontal health and prevent recurrence of attachment loss on a long-term basis (15 years) (Axelsson et al 1991). Can this be said of advanced periodontal disease? Some authors state that prognosis is inversely proportional to disease severity. This implies that a better prognosis is associated with mild forms of periodontitis, and, vice versa, that advanced forms of periodontitis are associated with a poor prognosis. However, this concept should be questioned. Attachment loss does not progress in a linear, continuous fashion, and it is not inevitable. Advanced forms of periodontitis require more periodontal therapy, more adjunctive treatments, and, more generally, more attention. When multidisciplinary care is carried out successfully, when response to treatment is favorable, when all the different risk factors have been taken into account, and when periodontal maintenance is efficient, periodontal health is likely to be maintained over very long periods (Fig 7-5).

Elimination of functional disorders (mobility, migrations) or periodontal defects (attachment loss, bone lesions) without resorting to adjunctive forms of treatment is a rare privilege and should be seized whenever possible.

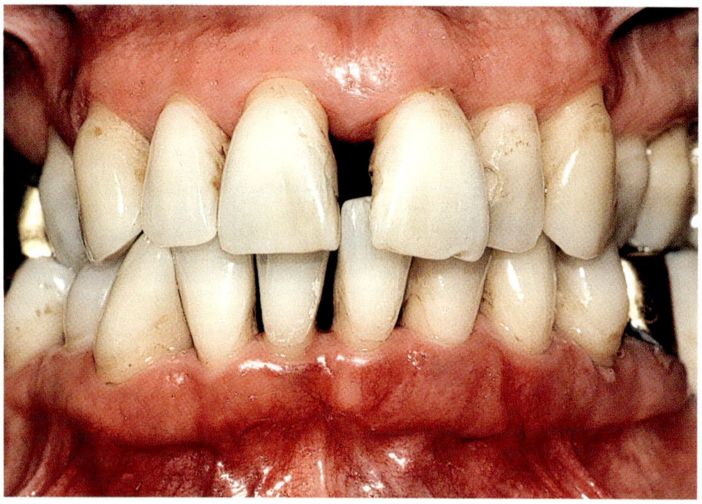

Fig 7-5a Advanced chronic periodontitis in a 45-year-old female patient. All usual signs of periodontitis are present: inflammation, mobility, migrations, diastemata, attachment loss, deep pockets, pain, and functional impairment.

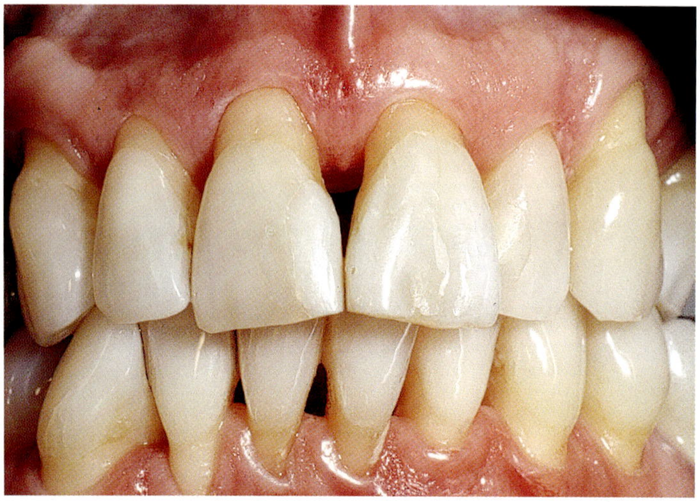

Fig 7-5b Sixteen years after periodontal treatment, all reversible signs of periodontitis, that is, inflammation, mobility, migrations, and diastemata, have disappeared. Partially reversible signs, including attachment losses, pockets, and bone destruction, have improved.

The periodontium has regained its functional dynamics. Clinicians have reliable evaluation criteria close at hand; these are precise and useful during periodontal maintenance and are also necessary before commencing rehabilitation. Rigid, nonmodifiable forms of rehabilitation, such as splinting devices and extensive prosthetic constructions, are not necessarily well-adapted to periodontal function. On the other hand, implant rehabilitation carries a better prognosis if periodontal function of remaining teeth is well maintained, and also if implant technology stands the test of time.

Glossary

Attachment gain Difference between the initial attachment level and the level obtained at the end of periodontal treatment.

Attachment level Distance between the cementoenamel junction and the bottom of the gingival sulcus or periodontal pocket, when inflammation is absent.

Attachment loss Difference between the ideal attachment level, before onset of disease, and the attachment level as observed in diseased periodontium. A renewed attachment loss is equivalent to the difference between both scores.

Bleeding on probing index (simplified) 0 = no bleeding on probing; 1 = presence of bleeding on probing.

Bone gain Difference between the initial bone level and the level obtained at the end of periodontal treatment; this is achieved through repair, grafting, or regeneration techniques.

Bone level Distance between the cementoenamel junction and the bone crest.

Bone loss (bone destruction) This is either horizontal, angular, or interradicular. Horizontal bone loss is evaluated in proportion to root length and is assessed radiographically using the horizontal planes technique, where the radiographic film is parallel to the sagittal plane of tooth.

Bony crater Superficial osseous lesion. The lesion is extended and shallow and is characterized by a poor capacity for repair. Bony craters are corrected by subtractive surgery, ie, osteoplasty.

Bony lesion (angular bone destruction) Characterized by width, depth, and number of environing walls. A slim, deep lesion presents a better potential for repair than a shallow, extended lesion.

Interradicular lesions
Class I Periodontal probe does not go beyond one third of the tooth's width.
Class II Periodontal probe goes beyond one third of the tooth's width.
Class III Periodontal probe is driven freely through the furcation.

New attachment Complete restoration of attachment system with new formation of bone, cementum, and connective fibers.

Probing The periodontal probe measures the propensity to bleeding on probing, pocket depth, and attachment level.

Probing depth/periodontal pocket depth Distance from the free gingival margin to the most apical part of the periodontal pocket.

Probing depth reduction/pocket depth reduction Difference between the pocket depth before and after treatment.

Reattachment Repair of attachment system, excluding any new formation of bone or cementum. This may involve the formation of a long junctional epithelium.

Simplified plaque index 0 = no plaque; 1 = presence of plaque.

Tooth mobility
Class I Physiologic mobility; intact periodontal tissue.
Class II Visible mobility; mobility of the tooth crown does not exceed 1 mm in amplitude.
Class III Crown mobility exceeds 1 mm.
Class IV Tooth presents mobility in a vertical direction.

Bibliography

Ainamo J, Barmes D, Beagrie G, Cutress T, Martin J, Sardo-Infirri J. Development of the World Health Organization (WHO) community periodontal index of treatment needs (CPITN). Int Dent J 1982;32:281–291.

Albandar JM, Brunelle JA, Kingman A. Destructive periodontal disease in adults 30 years of age and older in the United States, 1988–1994. J Periodontol 1999;70: 13–29.

American Academy of Periodontology. Parameters of care. J Periodontol 2000;71(suppl):847–883.

American Academy of Periodontology. Parameters of care. Parameter on plaque-induced gingivitis. J Periodontol 2000;71(suppl):851–852.

American Academy of Periodontology. Parameters of care. Parameter on chronic periodontitis with slight to moderate loss of periodontal support. J Periodontol 2000; 71(suppl):853–855.

American Academy of Periodontology. Parameters of care. Parameter on chronic periodontitis with advanced loss of periodontal support. J Periodontol 2000;71(suppl): 856–858.

American Academy of Periodontology. Parameters of care. Parameter on aggressive periodontitis. J Periodontol 2000;71(suppl):867–869.

American Academy of Periodontology. Parameters of care. Parameter on periodontal maintenance. J Periodontol 2000;71(suppl):849–883.

Armitage GC. Development of a classification system for periodontal diseases and conditions. Ann Periodontol 1999;4:1–6.

Axelsson P, Lindhe J, Nystrom B. On the prevention of caries and periodontal disease. Results of a 15-year longitudinal study in adults. J Clin Periodontol 1991;18: 182–189.

Axelsson P, Paulander J, Lindhe J. Relationship between smoking and dental status in 35-, 50-, 65-, and 75-year-old individuals. J Clin Periodontol 1998;25:297–305.

Badersten A, Nilveus R, Egelberg J. Effect of nonsurgical periodontal therapy. VII. Bleeding, suppuration and probing depth in sites with probing attachment loss. J Clin Periodontol 1985;12:432–440.

Baelum V, Fejerskov O, Manji F. Periodontal diseases in adult Kenyans. J Clin Periodontol 1988;15:445–452.

Beck J, Garcia R, Heiss G, Vokonas PS, Offenbacher S. Periodontal disease and cardiovascular disease. J Periodontol 1996;67(suppl):1123–1137.

Becker W, Becker BE, Ochsenbein C, et al. A longitudinal study comparing scaling, osseous surgery and modified Widman procedures. Results after one year. J Periodontol 1988;59:351–365.

Brecx MC, Lehmann B, Siegwart CM, Gehr P, Lang NP. Observations on the initial stages of healing following human experimental gingivitis. A clinical and morphometric study. J Clin Periodontol 1988;15:123–129.

Brown LJ, Oliver RC, Löe H. Periodontal diseases in the U.S. in 1981: Prevalence, severity, extent, and role in tooth mortality. J Periodontol 1989;60:363–370.

Caffesse RG, de la Rosa M, de la Rosa G. The role of IL-1 genotype on periodontal maintenance needs [abstract 263]. J Clin Periodontol 2000;27(S1).

Caffesse RG, Sweeney PL, Smith BA. Scaling and root planing with and without periodontal flap surgery. J Clin Periodontol 1986;13:205–210.

Camelo M, Nevins ML, Lynch SE, Schenk RK, Simion M, Nevins M. Periodontal regeneration with an autogenous bone–Bio-Oss composite graft and a Bio-Gide membrane. Int J Periodontics Restorative Dent 2001; 21:109–119.

Costerton JW, Lewandowski Z, DeBeer D, Caldwell D, Korber D, James G. Biofilms, the customized microniche. J Bacteriol 1994;176:2137–2142.

Craig RG, Boylan R, Yip J, et al. Prevalence and risk indicators for destructive periodontal diseases in 3 urban American minority populations. J Clin Periodontol 2001;28:524–535.

Dahlen G, Lindhe J, Sato K, Hanamura H, Okamoto H. The effect of supragingival plaque control on the subgingival microbiota in subjects with periodontal disease. J Clin Periodontol 1992;19:802–809.

Darveau RP, Tanner A, Page RC. The microbial challenge in periodontitis. Periodontol 2000 1997;14:12–32.

De Sanctis M, Zucchelli G. Interleukin-1 gene polymorphisms and long-term stability following guided tissue regeneration therapy. J Periodontol 2000;71:606–713.

Ebersole JL, Taubman MA. The protective nature of host responses in periodontal diseases. Periodontol 2000 1994;5:112–141.

Fardal O, Johannessen AC, Olsen I. Severe, rapidly progressing peri-implantitis. J Clin Periodontol 1999;26: 313–317.

Feres M, Haffajee AD, Allard K, Som S, Socransky SS. Change in subgingival microbial profiles in adult periodontitis subjects receiving either systemically administered amoxicillin or metronidazole. J Clin Periodontol 2001;28:597–609.

Feres M, Haffajee AD, Allard K, Som S, Goodson JM, Socransky SS. Antibiotic resistance of subgingival species during and after antibiotic therapy. J Clin Periodontol 2002;29:724–735.

Fleischer HC, Mellonig JT, Brayer WK, Gray JL, Barnett JD. Scaling and root planing efficacy in multirooted teeth. J Periodontol 1989;60:402–409.

Giargia M, Lindhe J. Tooth mobility and periodontal disease. J Clin Periodontol 1997;24:785–795.

Goodson JM. Antimicrobial strategies for treatment of periodontal diseases. Periodontol 2000 1994;5:142–168.

Griffiths GS, Wilton JM, Curtis MA, et al. Detection of high-risk groups and individuals for periodontal diseases: Clinical assessment of the periodontium. J Clin Periodontol 1988;15:403–410.

Grossi SG, Genco RJ, Machtei EE, et al. Assessment of risk for periodontal disease. II. Risk indicators for alveolar bone loss. J Periodontol 1995;66:23–29.

Grossi SG, Zambon JJ, Ho AW, et al. Assessment of risk for periodontal disease. I. Risk indicators for attachment loss. J Periodontol 1994;65:260–267.

Haffajee AD, Cugini MA, Dibart S, Smith C, Kent RL Jr, Socransky SS. The effect of SRP on the clinical and microbiological parameters of periodontal diseases. J Clin Periodontol 1997;24:324–34.

Haffajee AD, Socransky SS. Microbial etiological agents of destructive periodontal diseases. Periodontol 2000 1994; 5:78–111.

Haffajee AD, Socransky SS. Relationship of cigarette smoking to attachment level profiles. J Clin Periodontol 2001; 28:283–295.

Haffajee AD, Smith C, Torresyap G, Thompson M, Guerrero D, Socransky SS. Efficacy of manual and powered toothbrushes (II). Effect on microbiological parameters. J Clin Periodontol 2001;28:947–954.

Haffajee AD, Thompson M, Torresyap G, Guerrero D, Socransky SS. Efficacy of manual and powered toothbrushes (I). Effect on clinical parameters. J Clin Periodontol 2001;28:937–946.

Institut National de la Santé et de la Recherche Médicale. Maladies Parodontales: Thérapeutiques et Prevention. INSERM: Paris, 1999.

Ishikawa I, Nakashima K, Koseki T, et al. Induction of the immune response to periodontopathic bacteria and its role in the pathogenesis of periodontitis. Periodontol 2000 1997;14:79–111.

Johnson NW, Griffiths GS, Wilton JM, et al. Detection of high-risk groups and individuals for periodontal diseases. Evidence for the existence of high-risk groups and individuals and approaches to their detection. J Clin Periodontol 1988;15:276–282.

Kinane DF, Lindhe J. Pathogenesis of periodontal tissue. In: Lindhe J (ed). Textbook of Periodontology. Copenhagen: Munksgaard, 1997.

Kornman KS, Crane A, Wang HY, et al. The interleukin-1 genotype as a severity factor in adult periodontal disease. J Clin Periodontol 1997;24:72–77.

Kornman KS, Page RC, Tonetti MS. The pathogenesis of human periodontitis: An introduction. Periodontol 2000 1997;14:9–11.

Lang NP, Joss A, Orsanic T, Gusberti FA, Siegrist BE. Bleeding on probing. A predictor for the progression of periodontal disease? J Clin Periodontol 1986;13:590–596.

Levy RM, Giannobile WV, Feres M, Haffajee AD, Smith C, Socransky SS. The short-term effect of apically repositioned flap surgery on the composition of the subgingival microbiota. Int J Periodontics Restorative Dent 1999;19:555–567.

Lindhe J, Nyman S. The effect of plaque control and surgical pocket elimination on the establishment and maintenance of periodontal health. A longitudinal study of periodontal therapy in cases of advanced disease. J Clin Periodontol 1975;2:67–79.

Listgarten MA. Formation of dental plaque and other oral biofilms. In: Newman HN, Wilson M (eds). Dental Plaque Revisited: Oral Biofilms in Health and Disease. [Proceedings of a conference held at the Royal College of Physicians, 3–5 November 1999, London.]Cardiff, UK: BioLine, 1999.

Listgarten MA. The structure of dental plaque. Periodontol 2000 1994;5:52–65.

Listgarten MA, Slots J, Nowotny AH, et al. Incidence of periodontitis recurrence in treated patients with and without cultivable *Actinobacillus actinomycetemcomitans, Prevotella intermedia,* and *Porphyromonas gingivalis*: A prospective study. J Periodontol 1991;62:377–386.

Löe H, Anerud A, Boysen H, Morrison E. Natural history of periodontal disease in man. Rapid, moderate and no loss of attachment in Sri Lankan laborers 14 to 46 years of age. J Clin Periodontol 1986;13:431–445.

Loos B, Claffey N, Egelberg J. Clinical and microbiological effects of root debridement in periodontal furcation pockets. J Clin Periodontol 1988;15:453–463.

Loos B, Nylund K, Claffey N, Egelberg J. Clinical effects of root debridement in molar and non-molar teeth. A 2-year follow-up. J Clin Periodontol 1989;16:498–504.

McGuire MK, Nunn ME. Prognosis versus actual outcome. IV. The effectiveness of clinical parameters and IL-1 genotype in accurately predicting prognoses and tooth survival. J Periodontol 1999;70:49–56.

Mombelli A, Lang NP. Microbial aspects of implant dentistry. Periodontol 2000 1994;4:74–80.

Norderyd O, Hugoson A, Grusovin G. Risk of severe periodontal disease in a Swedish adult population. A longitudinal study. J Clin Periodontol 1999;26:608–615.

Nowzari H, MacDonald ES, Flynn J, London RM, Morrison JL, Slots J. The dynamics of microbial colonization of barrier membranes for guided tissue regeneration. J Periodontol 1996;67:694–702.

Nowzari H, Slots J. Microorganisms in polytetrafluoroethylene barrier membranes for guided tissue regeneration. J Clin Periodontol 1994;21:203–210.

Nyman S, Rosling B, Lindhe J. Effect of professional tooth cleaning on healing after periodontal surgery. J Clin Periodontol 1975;2:80–86.

Nyman S, Westfelt E, Sarhed G, Karring T. Role of "diseased" root cementum in healing following treatment of periodontal disease. A clinical study. J Clin Periodontol 1988;15:464–468.

Offenbacher S, Katz V, Fertik G, et al. Periodontal infection as a possible risk factor for preterm low birth weight. J Periodontol 1996;67(10 suppl):1103–1113.

Page RC, Offenbacher S, Schroeder HE, Seymour GJ, Kornman KS. Advances in the pathogenesis of periodontitis: Summary of developments, clinical implications and future directions. Periodontol 2000 1997;14:216–248.

Pavicic MJ, van Winkelhoff AJ, Douque NH, Steures RW, de Graaff J. Microbiological and clinical effects of metronidazole and amoxicillin in *Actinobacillus actinomycetemcomitans*-associated periodontitis. A 2-year evaluation. J Clin Periodontol 1994;21:107–112.

Quirynen M, Listgarten MA. Distribution of bacterial morphotypes around natural teeth and titanium implants ad modum Bränemark. Clin Oral Implants Res 1990;1:8–12.

Ramfjord SP, Caffesse RG, Morrison EC, et al. Four modalities of periodontal treatment compared over 5 years. J Clin Periodontol 1987;14:445–452.

Rawlinson A, Duerden BI, Goodwin L. Effects of surgical treatment on the microbial flora in residual periodontal pockets. Eur J Prosthodont Restor Dent 1995;3: 155–161.

Renvert S, Wikstrom M, Dahlen G, Slots J, Egelberg J. Effect of root debridement on the elimination of *Actinobacillus actinomycetemcomitans* and *Bacteroides gingivalis* from periodontal pockets. J Clin Periodontol 1990;17:345–350.

Renvert S, Wikstrom M, Dahlen G, Slots J, Egelberg J. On the inability of root debridement and periodontal surgery to eliminate *Actinobacillus actinomycetemcomitans* from periodontal pockets. J Clin Periodontol 1990;17:351–355.

Reynolds JJ, Meikle MC. Mechanisms of connective tissue matrix destruction in periodontitis. Periodontol 2000 1997;14:144–157.

Rosenberg ES, Evian CI, Listgarten MA. The composition of the subgingival microbiota after periodontal therapy. J Periodontol 1981;52:435–441.

Sayers NM, James JA, Drucker DB, Blinkhorn AS. Possible potentiation of toxins from *Prevotella intermedia, Prevotella nigrescens,* and *Porphyromonas gingivalis* by cotinine. J Periodontol 1999;70:1269–1275.

Sbordone L, Barone A, Ciaglia RN, Ramaglia L, Iacono VJ. Longitudinal study of dental implants in a periodontally compromised population. J Periodontol 1999;70:1322–1329.

Scabbia A, Cho KS, Sigurdsson TJ, Kim CK, Trombelli L. Cigarette smoking negatively affects healing response following flap debridement surgery. J Periodontol 2001; 72:43–49.

Schwartz Z, Goultschin J, Dean DD, Boyan BD. Mechanisms of alveolar bone destruction in periodontitis. Periodontol 2000 1997;14:158–172.

Serino G, Rosling B, Ramberg P, Socransky SS, Lindhe J. Initial outcome and long-term effect of surgical and non-surgical treatment of advanced periodontal disease. J Clin Periodontol 2001;28:910–916.

Sheiham A. Screening for periodontal disease. J Clin Periodontol 1978;5:237–245.

Sherman PR, Hutchens LH Jr, Jewson LG. The effectiveness of subgingival scaling and root planing. II. Clinical responses related to residual calculus. J Periodontol 1990;61:9–15.

Sigusch B, Beier M, Klinger G, Pfister W, Glockmann E. A 2-step non-surgical procedure and systemic antibiotics in the treatment of rapidly progressive periodontitis. J Periodontol 2001;72:275–283.

Slots J, Listgarten MA. *Bacteroides gingivalis, Bacteroides intermedius* and *Actinobacillus actinomycetemcomitans* in human periodontal diseases. J Clin Periodontol 1988;15:85–93.

Slots J, Ting M. *Actinobacillus actinomycetemcomitans* and *Porphyromonas gingivalis* in human periodontal disease: Occurrence and treatment. Periodontol 2000 1999;20:82–121.

Socransky SS, Haffajee AD. The bacterial etiology of destructive periodontal disease: Current concepts. J Periodontol 1992;63(4 suppl):322–331.

Socransky SS, Haffajee AD. Evidence of bacterial etiology: A historical perspective. Periodontol 2000 1994;5:7–25.

Socransky SS, Haffajee AD, Cugini MA, Smith C, Kent RL Jr. Microbial complexes in subgingival plaque. J Clin Periodontol 1998;25:134–144.

Socransky SS, Haffajee AD, Ximenez-Fyvie LA, Feres M, Mager D. Ecological considerations in the treatment of *Actinobacillus actinomycetemcomitans* and *Porphyromonas gingivalis* periodontal infections. Periodontol 2000 1999;20:341–362.

Socransky SS, Haffajee AD, Smith C, Duff GW. Microbiological parameters associated with IL-1 gene polymorphisms in periodontitis patients. J Clin Periodontol 2000;27:810–818.

Svardstrom G, Wennstrom JL. Periodontal treatment decisions for molars: An analysis of influencing factors and long-term outcome. J Periodontol 2000;71:579–585.

Timmerman MF, Van der Weijden GA, Arief EM, et al. Untreated periodontal disease in Indonesian adolescents. Subgingival microbiota in relation to experienced progression of periodontitis. J Clin Periodontol 2001;28:617–627.

Tuan MC, Nowzari H, Slots J. Clinical and microbiologic study of periodontal surgery by means of apically positioned flaps with and without osseous recontouring. Int J Periodontics Restorative Dent 2000;20:468–475.

van Winkelhoff AJ, Rams TE, Slots J. Systemic antibiotic therapy in periodontics. Periodontol 2000 1996;10:45–78.

van Winkelhoff AJ, Tijhof CJ, de Graaff J. Microbiological and clinical results of metronidazole plus amoxicillin therapy in *Actinobacillus actinomycetemcomitans*-associated periodontitis. J Periodontol 1992;63:52–57.

van Winkelhoff AJ, Wolf JW. *Actinobacillus actinomycetemcomitans*-associated peri-implantitis in an edentulous patient. A case report. J Clin Periodontol 2000;27: 531–535.

Waerhaug J. A method for evaluation of periodontal problems on extracted teeth. J Clin Periodontol 1975;2: 160–168.

Winkel EG, Van Winkelhoff AJ, Timmerman MF, Van der Velden U, Van der Weijden GA. Amoxicillin plus metronidazole in the treatment of adult periodontitis patients. A double-blind placebo-controlled study. J Clin Periodontol 2001;28:296–305.

Yuodelis RA, Faucher R. An integrated approach to periodontics and restorative dentistry. Dent Clin North Am 1980;24:285–303.

Index

Page numbers followed by "t" denote tables; those followed by "f" denote figures

Imprimé en France par EMD S.A.S - 53110 Lassay-les-Châteaux
N° d' imprimeur : 14313 - Dépôt légal : septembre 2005